OVERCOMING IMPOSTER SYNDROME:

YOU BELONG AT THE TABLE!

Anthony W. Scott, Esq.

I.S.I. Publishing LLC
P.O. Box 29037 Parma,
OH 44129
Email: info@isiconsultingllc.com
Website: www.isiconsultingllc.com

ISBN *(Paperback)*: 9798992015744
ISBN *(e-Book)*: 9798992015751

Edited by Chyina Powell with Powell Editorial
Foreword by Dr. Anthony Redic, Organizational Psychology
First Edition
Printed in the United States of America

This book is a work of nonfiction. While every effort has been made to ensure accuracy, the author and publisher assume no responsibility for errors, omissions, or contrary interpretation of the subject matter contained herein.

For bulk order discounts, special inquiries or to request Anthony W. Scott, Esq. for a speaking engagement, please contact info@isiconsultingllc.com.

DEDICATION

To My Village-thank you for pouring into my cup, allowing it to overflow. Without y'all I wouldn't have been able to have written this book; I would still be too deeply immersed in my own Imposter Syndrome.

To those Brave Souls that allowed me to interview them for this book. Thank you for sharing your time, your stories, your struggles and your growth with us. You know who you are (shhh...I won't tell).

...And, as always, "Showt Owt" to my Beloved Wife, Carmen Milagro Scott—My Muse. I'm still head over heels in love with you because of your continued love, support, encouragement, patience and tolerance as WE continue on this A-Maz-Ing adventure called The Scotts.

FOREWORD

The thief comes only to steal, kill, and destroy... (John 10:10).

Imposter syndrome is like a thief, and it has robbed and destroyed many confident voices, amazing dreams, wild ambitions, and written goals. Accomplished professionals can't find peace and aspiring leaders can't find their worth. Those who live at the intersectionality of race, class, gender, and identity have watched, in real-time, the thief use doubt, uncertainty, and self-suspicion to erode what confidences they have left. Even the tables we've earned seats at seem uncomfortable and wobbly because of the voices in our own heads. Imposter Syndrome is a real enemy that must be dealt with!

Like a skilled surgeon using a scalpel to perform a delicate procedure, Anthony W. Scott, Esq., has shined a light on this seemingly invisible disease. With brutal honesty, cultural understanding, and an unrelenting desire to tell the whole truth, he has revealed the mystery of this plague. His personal story, and the stories of others within these chapters, are like a mirror and medicine. A mirror because it reflects the quiet suffering so many of us carry on a daily basis. Medicine because it offers validation of our experiences and hope for a future with a different internal narrative.

This book is set apart, not only because of its vulnerability, but also because of its insight, education, and a way forward. Scott reminds us that this disease does not operate in isolation...it is deeply rooted in systemic bias, cultural expectations, and childhood survival strategies. If you've ever been told that you have to be "twice as good" this book is a must read.

This book had me locked in from the very beginning because I could relate. I was even transported back to a past situation...a specific meeting where I, now know, imposter syndrome was present and won that day. I get angry thinking about it...

> *I was working for a fortune 100 company, and I had to present to my leadership on a process challenge. As is often the case, I was the only Black Man in the room, (there was a Black female in attendance as well). I understood the issue and was well-prepared. I was not surprised how well the presentation went (I was prepared), and I led the discussion as the knowledgeable expert I was. As we began to discuss solutions, several questions were raised, and assumptions were made. I HAD THE RIGHT SOLUTION! BUT I KEPT QUIET. A few moments later, a colleague spoke up and shared the same idea that I had...I was mortified! The room buzzed with excitement and my colleague was acknowledged for their insightfulness and analysis. I stood in front of the room, trying hard to maintain a stoic facial expression, but on the inside, I was sick.*

This is why, I know, this book, *Overcoming Imposter Syndrome*, is a godsend. Through research, honest talk, and raw experiences, you will be armed with a new blueprint and battle strategy. Whether you are a corporate executive, a community leader, a student, a changemaker, or someone who simply wants to be more comfortable in their own skin...this book is absolutely for you. In it, you will find where you are and where you were meant to be.

So, grab *Overcoming Imposter Syndrome*, (and some paper for note taking), pull up a chair, put your elbows on the table, get comfortable, and know...YOU BELONG!

Dr. Anthony B. Redic

Organizational Psychology

Contents

INTRODUCTION

YOU ARE NOT ALONE

Understanding Imposter Syndrome: A Universal Struggle

Imposter syndrome is not just self-doubt. It is an ongoing fear of being exposed as a fraud. It is a belief that no matter how much you accomplish, you are only one mistake away from being "found out." It whispers that your achievements aren't real. It sometimes screams "YOU DON'T BELONG", in these spaces you occupy. It nudges you into believing that, somehow, you've deceived the people who believe in you.

It's the feeling of walking into a boardroom, a courtroom, an operating room, or a high-profile meeting and thinking, *what if today is the day they realize I have no idea what I'm doing?* It's hearing someone introduce you with accolades and titles, only to think to yourself, *who are they talking about? That's not me.*

This struggle isn't unique to one group of people or one profession. It crosses industries, backgrounds, and identities. It affects executives, educators, artists, scientists, and students alike. Maya Angelou once said, "I have written eleven books, but each time I think, *Uh-oh,*

1

they're going to find me out now."[i] Even Albert Einstein, despite revolutionizing modern science, described himself as an "involuntary swindler," convinced people had overestimated his intelligence.[ii]

If you have ever felt like you don't deserve your success, that you're just lucky, or that you need to work twice as hard to prove you belong—you are not alone. I know this because I've lived it too.

Why This Book Matters

Imposter syndrome isn't new to me. I first explored the topic in my book *Unlocking Potential: Insights, Tips, and Strategies for Young Black Professionals*. I included it as a chapter because it kept showing up in my mentees, in my peers, and even within myself. But I knew before I had finished that book that a single chapter would not do the topic justice.

Imposter syndrome is present in most of us whether we realize it or not. It cannot be summarized in a few pages. It's more than a professional inconvenience. It is an anchor that limits our growth, regardless of how much evidence of credentials, qualifications, skills and success we have on paper. I have lived with that contradiction for most of my life. On the surface, humbly speaking, I've checked some impressive boxes. I am a United States Marine Corps veteran, a college graduate with a Bachelors, Masters, and Law Degree, an Attorney, a Director level government administrator, an author, and a business owner. However, beneath it all, my imposter syndrome still echoes quite LOUDLY at times.

This book is, in part, my unpacking how imposter syndrome has impacted my life. More importantly, it is an exploration of others who are fighting this same battle. Some stories show great progress and transformation. Others are still on their journey, writing their own chapters daily.

The Stories Behind the Science

As I began writing, I spoke with a diverse group of professionals from across the country that consisted of attorneys, healthcare providers, corporate executives, entrepreneurs and educators. They were composed of younger, older, male, female, Black, Hispanic, Caucasian, heterosexual and homosexual individuals. Some were eager to tell their stories. Others shared hesitantly, only after being assured their names would not be used. A few asked that their voices not be recorded at all.

So, I made a decision. I would change all their names and identifying details, even for those who gave me permission. I wanted to create a level playing field between those who felt they could speak freely and those who did not. I wanted to assure them that it was a safe space that allowed them to be open and vulnerable. I needed the authentic version of them, so I could show readers that imposter syndrome doesn't discriminate.

Their voices appear throughout this book. Sometimes in passing, sometimes as full narratives. Each one reveals something raw, honest, and deeply human about how imposter syndrome shows up in the real world. This monster shows up in hospital wings, board meetings, university classrooms, family dinner tables, and even lonely hotel rooms on the night before a big presentation.

If you see yourself in some of these stories, then my plan worked.

Who This Book Is For

The truth is, imposter syndrome doesn't care about your résumé. It doesn't vanish with a promotion or a degree. If anything, it becomes more pronounced the more successful you become. The higher you rise, the more you fear the fall. That fear affects:

- ➲ "High Achievers;"
- ➲ First-generation professionals navigating unfamiliar spaces;
- ➲ People of color, women, LGBTQIA+ individuals, and others underrepresented in positions of power; and,
- ➲ Anyone who's ever been "the only" or "the first" in the room.

If that resonates with you, I want you to know this...you are not broken. You are not alone. And you are NOT a FRAUD!

What This Book Seeks to Do

This book is not just a collection of psychological research. It's a blend of lived stories and real strategies. It offers insight, not from a wealth of research or studies, but from the people I interviewed and from myself. People that, despite impressive accomplishments, still struggle with the quiet belief that they are somehow not enough.

Each chapter connects these stories to the psychological and neurological realities behind imposter syndrome. While I am not a clinician, I've drawn on respected research and literature to frame what so many of us already know about ourselves. Our self-doubt is not always logical; but, it is deeply real.

Here's what you'll find in the pages ahead:

- ⮱ Why high achievers often feel the least confident;
- ⮱ How early life, identity, and systems of oppression shape our inner critics;
- ⮱ The science of self-doubt: how our brains misinterpret success as danger;
- ⮱ Why some people never feel "ready" and how to move forward anyway; and,
- ⮱ Practical tools to quiet the noise, stop the spiral, and take back control.

What this book will not do is promise a quick fix. This is not about waking up one day and never doubting yourself again. It's about learning to live with doubt in a way that doesn't sabotage your potential.

Further, it gives you a sense of community. Seeing yourself in others that have had, and still have, the same struggles as you is valuable. It reminds us that we also can rise above the insecurities that plague us and grow to greater heights personally and in our careers.

A Journey Toward Self-Acceptance

Imposter syndrome does not mean you are incompetent. Far from it. It means you have been conditioned by upbringing, culture, bias and/or by your own impossible standards. This conditioning has caused you to believe you must earn your place through perfection. You have been conditioned to believe that you are not enough and that you do not belong at "the table."

What is the table, you ask? The table is where decisions are made and voices are heard. It's a place of influence, leadership, visibility, and power. It's the meeting where strategy is shaped, the courtroom where outcomes are decided, the classroom where ideas are validated. The table is any space where your presence isn't just noticed, it changes the dynamic. It's a space where people like us haven't always been welcomed. And yet, we have arrived.

Overcoming imposter syndrome isn't about being fearless. It's about moving forward anyway. It's about building confidence through action, compassion, and a willingness to redefine success. Success defined by your own rules, not by other people's definitions.

So if you've ever felt like an imposter in your own life, this book is for you.

Your success is real and your story matters. Now it is time that you start believing it.

Next: My Story—Living with Imposter Syndrome

Before we go deeper into the experiences of others, I want to share my own. The next chapter is my personal reflection on how imposter syndrome has shaped, and continues to shape, my path. This will be the most honest assessment I have ever written as to how it began, it's evolved, and how I continue to navigate it today. My hope is that in telling my truth, you'll find pieces of your own. That you will also begin to rewrite the story that imposter syndrome has tried to tell you.

PART I

UNDERSTANDING IMPOSTER SYNDROME

Chapter 1

My Story

Introduction: Growing Up in East Cleveland, Ohio

I always joke that before I would ever consider running for a political office, I would tell my story. Like Eminem in *Eight Mile*, I am going to clown myself before anyone else gets a chance. To be clear, I have no intention of running for office, but, after this book, who knows. So, here it goes...

I was born in Cleveland, Ohio, but grew up in East Cleveland, Ohio. Poverty, drugs, and violence were part of daily life. I was my mother's only child, but my "sperm donor" had a few other kids that I never met (then again, I never remember meeting him either). I would not remember what he even looked like except for I used to be able to see his image on the Ohio Offender Database.

When I was very young, my mother married Russell Williams Sr. We had a difficult relationship as I was growing up and even, somewhat, as an adult. For years, I had a scar on my neck where the zipper on my sweatshirt cut me when he was choking me with it. He had struck my mom and I pounced on him. I might have been nine or ten years old. I think that was what prompted my mom to throw him out the first time, and let him back in for the first of many more times.

He did get better after they got divorced and remarried. I think that was when I was in 9th grade. He was the closest I ever had to a father figure and have loved, respected and feared him as such. I got my work ethic from him. Honestly, I was a momma's boy before he came along with his version of tough love. But for him, however, I would NOT be the man that I am today. Thanks Pops!

Along with Russell Sr. came by step-brother, Russell Jr. Mom, Pops and Junior have all passed away at this point.

One night stands out clearly. I once climbed out of a second-story window to go next door and have the neighbors call the police. The downstairs neighbor was drunk (or high). He and his wife were arguing about something, and it made its way upstairs to our apartment. I don't recall the reason, but he was holding my parents and his wife at gunpoint. When I heard the scuffle, I came out of my room and saw it. Russell Sr., hollered, "Go back in your room, Tony." So I did.

But instead of staying put, I tied two sheets together like they do in the movies. Russell Jr. tied the sheets to the steam radiator and tossed them out the window for me. I climbed down, only for the two sheets to come loose. I crashed to the ground, landing in the "sticker bushes" to break my fall. I didn't have time to lay there in pain. I had to get next door. Thankfully, the police came, no one was hurt, and the families went back to normal whenever he was released from jail.

That was East Cleveland for you. Before I ever learned to fight for my country as a United States Marine, I had already been fighting just to survive. I recall getting chased home after a Shaw and Glenville football game. Once the bullets started flying we all got separated as we ran through backyards, hopped fences, and hid. Stories like this were common for people I grew up with. People with crazy stories like this do not go on to live successful lives, at least that was my belief.

The Hustle for Legitimacy: Education, Survival, and Self-Doubt

I was the first in my family to graduate from college. My mom attended Cuyahoga Community College for a few semesters, but did not get a degree. I do not recall if either Russell Sr. or Jr. ever obtained their G.E.D. There was no roadmap for me. Every step forward felt like an experiment, a risk, and a test I was sure I would fail.

Even as I passed my classes and advanced, the self doubt lingered. I wanted to be an attorney when I was growing up but didn't think I was smart enough to pursue it. I only saw glimpses of being smart, even though I was in Honors classes. All of my friends were smarter and better than me in my mind. I failed 9th-grade English and had to attend summer school. I attended Upward Bound (UB), a college prep program for low income and first generation students. It's quite ironic that I had to quit UB

11

the following year. Since I failed English, I had to attend summer school to catch up.

I went to Cleveland State University on a scholarship but failed out in one semester since I was too busy chasing women and drinking—not studying, not attending class. So, I enlisted in the United States Marine Corps from 1990 to 1998, serving during Desert Storm/Desert Shield.

By God's Grace I was never on the ground in combat. Most of my time was spent in my MOS (Military Occupational Specialist) of 0121, Service Record Book Clerk. Thankfully, I tested into a MOS that did not drop me directly into combat. However, as luck would have it, I would get attached to an aircraft carrier, CVN-71, which was in the Middle East during the war for almost eighteen months over three different deployments. Thanks to those eight (8) years of service (including that time on the aircraft carrier) my anxiety, stress disorder, anger management are all present to this day. More about that later.

Resilience, Redemption, and the Path to Law

Once I did return home after my Honorable Discharge, I resumed my education. College was nothing special for me. It took me forever to graduate because I was working as many as three jobs at one time to make ends meet. Like Ice Cube in *Higher Learning*, I was a "Super Duper Senior."

I did whatever it took to pay for school. I would show up to class exhausted, running on caffeine and sheer determination, knowing that failure was not an option.

There was no safety net for me. Like I said, I worked multiple jobs. I remember working at Kmart as security. I worked as a personal trainer, a bouncer, and a bartender. I worked at a daycare center and eventually made my way into the world of customer service positions.

I must admit that I even worked as an exotic dancer for many years. I actually became decent at it before I eventually quit in graduate school. My stage name was "Creme" and I spent a few years with both Zeus and Rumpshaker's Crews (Appreciate you Harrison and Bobby).

Finally, it happened. I graduated. It took me a total of thirteen years from the day I graduated Shaw High School in 1990 to the day I graduated Cleveland State University with my Bachelor's Degree in English. And what did I do with that prestigious college degree? I went to work at a well known "Rent-A-Car" company.

I hated it, but I had bills to pay. I knew I wanted more, but I did not think I could accomplish more. Thankfully, that nagging feeling of "what if" would not leave me. Moreso, I had a village, just like when I was that kid in East Cleveland, that kept telling me I was destined for more.

So, I decided to apply to law school. I applied but did not get in. For three days, I sat at home and felt sorry for myself, playing Sega Genesis (for those too young to know, it predated Xbox and PlayStation). I didn't shower, shave, or exercise. I just played my game and ate pizza. After that brief pity party, I entered graduate school to improve my GPA, get a more expansive network for better reference letters. I re-applied to law school as soon as they started accepting applications. I did not realize how smart that was at the time. Turns out, the earlier I applied, the less competition there was for slots still open.

I had a 3.8 GPA when I reapplied to law school...and was accepted.

My grades were decent my first year. I secured a good job at the U.S. Attorney General's office. They asked me back, which was a clear indication of having done a good job. I turned it down to accept an internship in the office of then Cuyahoga County Commissioner, Peter Lawson-Jones, Esq. I gained invaluable experience in his office, learning how to navigate politics and high-profile positions.

The Evidence Was Stacked Against Me

When people hear that I started my own law firm, they often assume it was the natural next step. A power move. The kind of thing a driven, confident attorney does to expand their reach and lead on their own terms.

But that's not how it happened.

The truth is, I started my firm because I had nowhere else to go.

My first two legal jobs out of law school didn't just end badly, they ended in ways that shook my identity. They left me questioning whether I belonged in this profession at all.

Let me rewind a few years earlier for context. I was quite fortunate. In my 2nd year of law school, I had landed one of the most coveted roles a law student could hope for. I was hired as a summer associate at a respected law firm. In fact, I had three or four job offers.

If firms like you after that summer, you may receive a full time job offer upon graduation and successful passage of the Bar Exam. That summer went well and I did receive that coveted offer. Six figure salary, suits and cufflinks right out of law school. I was beyond pumped for the opportunity, but immediately questioned myself silently. On paper, it should've felt like affirmation. Proof that I was on the right path. But even as I accepted the offer, I remember thinking: *Why do they want me? They only want me because I'm Black. Because I'm a Marine. Because they think I'll be disciplined and easy to manage.*

Not because I'm smart, talented or I belong in this world.

Imposter syndrome was already seated beside me at the table, translating every compliment into a conditional clause. *"You did well...for someone like you." "You're impressive, but let's see if you can keep it up."* It didn't matter how genuine the praise sounded. By the time it reached me, it had been filtered through a voice in my head that demanded perfection and distrusted approval. Even in moments of recognition, I was scanning the room, wondering when someone would raise their hand and say, *"Actually, he doesn't belong here."*

That firm? I never really fit in. Some of it was my own doing. Imposter syndrome had created a self-fulfilling prophecy. I would not make it here. The rest of it, honestly, was because I did not actually fit in. I was one of only two Black attorneys, and there were no Hispanic attorneys. The one Black attorney became a great mentor. But we didn't work in the same areas, so she could only shepherd my career but so far. She did try though. Thank you Judge Jessica Price-Smith. You are STILL one of my heroes.

The assignments they gave me were uninspiring—grind work, not growth work. In hindsight, I know that is part of the evolution of a young associate. I hadn't matured yet, either. My personal life was a mess. My mother was spiraling with her mental health. I was drinking too much. My relationships were imploding. I was coming to work, but I wasn't *showing up*.

Still, I wasn't prepared for it to end.

They let me resign. They gave me a severance package that, at the time, felt like a consolation prize for failure. Two years in, and I was already stepping away from what I thought was going to be my big legal career.

Then came the second job. It was even more short-lived and even more discouraging. I lasted about six months. I'll never forget the day the Executive Director, a woman who had held that role for twenty-four years, pulled me aside and told me, "You should probably start looking for something very soon." I was smart enough to know I wouldn't win that fight, so I resigned that same month even though I had not found another job. I did not want a termination on my record.

Two jobs. Two exits. Less than three years.

That voice inside me, the one that had been whispering *you're not cut out for this*, became louder.

> *You're not meant for this profession. You're too messy. Too flawed. Too emotional. Too Black. Too loud. Too quiet. Too much, yet not enough.*

And to be honest, I wasn't getting a lot of callbacks. My résumé looked sharp. My interviews were solid (at least in my mind). But inside, I felt hollow. Unanchored. Disconnected from the very identity I had fought so hard to build.

So I did the only thing I could think of, I started my own firm...not because I had a grand business plan or a stack of clients lined up. Not because I was ready. I had bills to pay and mouths to feed, it was that simple.

Will the Shoe Drop?

Fast forward to today. As of this writing, I have been working for the City of Cleveland, Ohio for the last thirteen years. I do not practice law in my 9-5 anymore. My roles have changed, my paycheck has increased and, humbly, I have become an exponentially better leader. I have had a staff of over 500 people in one of my roles. That was a hell of a learning lesson! I manage staff at various levels of leadership and programs, including, ironically, an attorney. It is my job to pour into them and to help lead them to successful careers. I echo "*I cannot afford to be off my game*" to myself daily. My physical and mental health have to be better, which they are, albeit some of that is based on the meds that I am on. Nonetheless, I am better.

Outside my 9–5, I run I.S.I. Consulting LLC (named from Proverbs 27:17: *As iron sharpens iron, so one man sharpens another).* I support small businesses and nonprofit organizations with legal formation, operational structure, compliance, governance, and long-term sustainability. I also work with professionals with their personal and professional career development. The work is quite fulfilling. In many ways, it is an extension of who I've become. I am someone who doesn't just lead from position, but from purpose.

I had the audacity to write and publish a book, *Unlocking Potential: Insights, Tips & Strategies for Young Black Professionals.* Hopefully you purchased a copy, liked it and gave it a great review. If not, it is still on sale, so pick up a copy. Please and thank you.

In June I received an award from the Black Law Student Association for the Cleveland State University School of Law. My speech was well received. I actually received a standing ovation. I even sold a few books.

This upcoming week should be good as well. I believe I have three different events or presentations this week. I am, admittedly, riding high during this surreal moment in time.

Yet I am still worried, in those quiet moments, of the shoe dropping. *Will they figure out that I am a fraud?*

Changing the Narrative: Embracing the Journey

The reality is that I know I belong (*on most days at least*). So do you! Not because we are perfect. Not because we never struggled. Not because we have checked all the "right" boxes. We belong because we have earned it. We just have to embrace it and push past those quiet voices in our head that make us question, *do we really belong here?*

This book is about changing the narrative—for myself, for you, and for anyone who has ever felt like they weren't enough. A friend of mine who knows most of my story has said I have been through some of everything. I suppose that is accurate. I tend to take it for granted that I have endured and overcome many things. The reality is, I tend to think I am nothing special.

But the truth is, surviving East Cleveland, the military, mental health challenges, law school and the legal profession have made me resilient and resourceful. The hustle for legitimacy doesn't end with success; it ends when you finally accept that you belong, not despite your past but because of it.

If I can find my place, so can you.

Chapter 2

Origins of Imposter Syndrome

Introduction: The Persistent Fear of Being Found Out

First off, you will notice quite a few definitions and citations in this section. Don't worry, there won't be a quiz. But, these terms matter because you'll see them again throughout the book. They don't exist in isolation; many overlap, build on one another, and compound the weight of imposter syndrome. This experience is more than just self-doubt. It is an unrelenting belief that your success isn't legitimate. You feel as if you've somehow deceived others into thinking you're more capable than you truly are. The fear of being exposed as a fraud lurks beneath each accomplishment. *Will the shoe drop today?* That anxiety follows you, even in the face of overwhelming evidence that you've earned your place.

For many, especially those who've had to fight for every opportunity, imposter syndrome doesn't feel like a "cognitive distortion;" it feels like a survival skill. A cognitive distortion is an irrational, exaggerated thought pattern that fuels negative emotions.[iii] These patterns often take root automatically and distort reality in ways that reinforce fear, insecurity, and self-doubt. When society has continually suggested, both subtly and explicitly, that certain spaces weren't made for you, it's hard *not* to internalize that narrative. Still, imposter syndrome is a learned response, not a fixed truth. The more we understand how these patterns are formed, the better equipped we are to dismantle them. Then we can reclaim the confidence we were meant to have in the first place.

Why High Achievers Are Most at Risk

Ironically, the more successful you are, the more likely you might feel like an imposter. That's because truly skilled people are often very aware of what they *don't* know. This self-awareness can make them feel inadequate, even when others see them as confident and capable. There's a disconnect between how they see themselves and how the world sees them.

This can be explained by the "Dunning-Kruger Effect"—a bias where people with low skill levels tend to overestimate their ability.[iv] Meanwhile, highly skilled people often underestimate their abilities.[v] The more someone knows, the more aware they are of what they don't know. That awareness can make them feel like others are more confident, capable, or deserving, even when that's not true. Think of the movie, *Dumb and Dumber* and how many times they thought that everyone else in the cast was the clueless person. That is Dunning-Kreuger.

Another psychological element at play is cognitive dissonance. Cognitive dissonance is the discomfort that arises when an individual holds two conflicting beliefs, such as *"I am successful"* and *"I don't deserve this success.* [vi] To resolve this conflict, the mind often rejects the positive belief, convincing you that your achievements must be a fluke. Or, they are the result of having deceived others rather than evidence of your capabilities. These competing perspectives allow imposter syndrome to persist, making it nearly impossible to internalize success as earned and deserved.

The Role of Comparison Culture in Reinforcing Self-Doubt

Comparison culture is the habit of constantly measuring yourself against others—how they look, what they've achieved, or how their lives appear—especially on social media. We called it "keeping up with the Joneses" when I was young. This often leads to feelings of inadequacy because people compare their real lives to others' "highlight reels." [vii] We are annoyingly connected in today's world. Social media and our professional networks can broadcast a never-ending stream of achievements. It is, unfortunately, easy to fall into this trap.

You have to remember that what you see are the polished highlights of others' lives. You cannot look at just the accolades, the promotions, and the successes without comparing them to the struggles, setbacks, or failures. That view lacks reality and perspective. It creates an illusion of effortless success that makes your own achievements feel smaller, your doubts more legitimate, and your struggles proof of unworthiness.

Anthony W. Scott

Admittedly, I sometimes look at my own social media as if I am looking at someone else. As an entrepreneur, I embrace the need to publicize my business on social media. Even though they are my accomplishments, events or thoughts, I do not always recognize them. The cognitive dissonance does not always allow me to recognize myself.

When all you see are the results and never the late nights, the failures, or the countless revisions, it is easy to conclude that you are the only one who feels uncertain. The visibility of success, contrasted with the invisibility of struggle, is fertile soil for imposter syndrome. The more you compare yourself to others' curated realities, the more convinced you become that your success is somehow fraudulent.

The Trap of Perfectionism and Fear of Failure

Imposter syndrome does not exist in a vacuum. It is heavily commingled with perfectionism. Perfectionism leaves you with the feeling that you always have to get everything exactly right. And if you don't, you feel like you've failed. It's more than wanting to do well, it's tying your self-worth to being flawless.[viii] People who struggle with perfectionism often fear making mistakes, are hard on themselves, and may avoid challenges just to dodge failure. Perfectionists tend to believe that anything short of perfection is failure and that success only counts if it is achieved independently and with great difficulty.[ix] This "all-or-nothing mentality" leaves no room for progress, learning, or self-compassion. Success is never enough, and failure is not an option.[x]

This mindset creates a vicious cycle. The more you achieve, the higher you raise the standard. Thereby, you inadvertently ensure that you never feel like you've truly earned your success. No matter how far you advance, it never feels like enough. You minimize each new accomplishment, or worse, dismiss it entirely. It's like chasing a finish line that keeps moving.

How Cognitive Distortions Fuel Imposter Syndrome

At its core, cognitive distortions are what fuel our imposter syndrome. They distort how we interpret our abilities, achievements, and self-worth. They create mental filters that magnify flaws, minimize wins, and convince us that we are one mistake away from being exposed. However, because they often operate automatically, we rarely stop to question them.[xi]

All or Nothing Thinking:

All-or-nothing thinking is a common cognitive distortion among high achievers. There is no middle ground. You either triumph or defeat. Either you are flawless or you are a failure. Remember what Ricky Bobby's dad taught him in *Talladega Nights,* "if you're not first your last." This kind of thinking leaves no room for growth, learning, or progress. It forces individuals into a perpetual state of dissatisfaction. When perfection is the only acceptable standard, even substantial achievements feel inadequate, and the smallest mistake feels like a disaster. Again, look at Ricky Bobby's life once he started losing races—he cracked completely (no spoiler alerts, go watch it if you have not seen it).

This mindset is often rooted in childhood experiences where praise was given for perfect performance rather than effort or progress. Children that were awarded solely for straight A's or winning sports competitions, rather than for trying hard or learning new skills, internalize the belief that anything less than perfection is failure. This pattern carries into adulthood. Every achievement is dissected for flaws and every mistake feels like an indictment of worth.

In professional settings, all-or-nothing thinking manifests as an unwillingness to delegate tasks, avoidance of risks that might expose gaps in knowledge, and a constant need for external validation.[xii] For example, a marketing executive might hesitate to propose a new campaign for fear that any imperfection could damage their credibility. Instead they opt for safer but less impactful projects. Similarly, a lawyer might refuse to take on complex cases that would expand their skills because the risk of making a mistake feels too high.

The real danger of all-or-nothing thinking is that it prevents growth. When perfection is the baseline, there is no room for experimentation, risk-taking, or the incremental progress that is necessary for real success. This mindset leads to avoidance behaviors—procrastination, refusal to delegate tasks, or an unwillingness to pursue new opportunities—because anything less than perfection feels like incompetence.

To shift this mindset, it's important to recognize that success exists on a spectrum. It is not always a win or lose scenario. Reshape your perspective. Partial successes, incremental improvements, and lessons learned are valid forms of progress that help disrupt the all-or-nothing mindset.

Catastrophizing:

Another common mental trap is catastrophizing. This essentially means that we blow small mistakes way out of proportion. If you miss a deadline, stumble during a presentation, or get constructive feedback, your mind spirals:. *"I've ruined everything." "They're going to realize I don't belong here." "This is the beginning of the end."*

Catastrophizing turns everyday bumps in the road into full-blown disasters, at least in your mind. That one slip-up isn't just a mistake. It becomes "proof" that all your success has been a fluke and that your exposure as a fraud is inevitable. This kind of thinking doesn't just hurt your confidence. It creates a paralyzing fear of failure that keeps you quiet when you should speak up, stagnant when you should take risks, and stuck in cycles of overthinking and regret.

Psychologists link catastrophizing to anxiety and imposter syndrome, noting it reinforces a constant state of threat, whether real or not.[xiii] Over time, catastrophizing echoes that same fear of failure we discussed with perfectionism. It is best to stay safe and in your small "bubble" that you know. If you stay in it, you are safe. Nothing can be taken from you. You cannot be harmed.

You cannot be found out as a fake. The truth is, making mistakes doesn't make you a fraud, it makes you human.

Discounting Achievements:

There is the habit, often unconscious, of discounting your own achievements. You hit a milestone, get the job, ace the interview, or receive praise. Instead of feeling proud, you downplay it. *"They must have had low expectations." "I just got lucky." "If they really knew me, they'd see I don't deserve this."* Sound familiar? This isn't humility. It is a cognitive distortion that rewrites your accomplishments as flukes or frauds, rather than the result of your hard work, skill, and resilience.

Psychologists call this success attribution bias, a pattern where individuals attribute success to external factors like luck, timing, or others' lowered expectations. They blame failure on internal flaws.[xiv] It's one of the core features of imposter syndrome. It creates a mental barrier that prevents you from truly owning your achievements. Even when you succeed, you don't feel successful. Instead of building confidence, each win is dismissed. You create a cycle where no amount of accomplishment is enough to silence your self-doubt. Over time, this can erode self-esteem and feed anxiety. Every new opportunity feels like another chance to be "found out."

But here's the truth, sometimes luck, your network, and even nepotism might open a door. However, it's your preparation, your persistence, and your presence that keep you in the room. *Well, maybe not if you are the boss' kid, but otherwise it's true...*

Breaking Free from Imposter Syndrome

To dismantle imposter syndrome, you must start by recognizing these cognitive distortions and actively challenging them. Reframe your achievements as earned rather than luck. Embrace progress over perfection. View failure as a part of growth rather than proof of inadequacy. It requires shifting from a mindset of proving your worth to one of owning your worth.

Imposter syndrome may never disappear entirely, but it can be managed. The goal is not to eliminate self-doubt but to learn how to act in spite of it. *How do we acknowledge it without letting it dictate our actions or define our worth?*

The next chapters will explore concrete strategies to silence the inner critic, embrace imperfection, and redefine success on your own terms.

The story of Isabella Vargas exemplifies the havoc these concepts can wreak on a young professional.

Growing Up in Athens, Ohio: Am I Enough for Any of Them?

Isabella Vargas (Izzy) was born in Lorain, Ohio, but spent much of her childhood in Athens, Ohio—a town of contrasts. On one side were the leafy streets and historic buildings of Ohio University. It was busy with professors, doctors, and students who seemed to embody the "American Dream." On the other side were the rows of nearly identical houses, subsidized by HUD,[xv] where Isabella and her family lived.

Her mixed heritage—Mexican from her mother's side and Puerto Rican from her father's—added another layer of complexity. As an Afro-Latina, Izzy constantly faced an unspoken question: *Am I enough for any of them?*

At school, she was one of the only Latinas. She was often mistaken for being Black, sometimes dismissed as "not really Latina" because her Spanish wasn't perfect. On visits to Lorain, her grandfather would remind her, "You're more than 50% Mexican," as if her identity could be weighed and measured. His words were meant to anchor her, but instead, they deepened her confusion. *If I'm more than 50% Mexican, does that make me less Puerto Rican?*

Financial Hardship's Emotional Toll: How Much Is Enough to Make It Worth It?

Growing up, Izzy's life was a delicate balance between survival and shame. Financial hardship was not just a reality; it was a reminder that every dollar spent needed justification. The fridge at home was often filled with basics—rice, beans, a few wilted vegetables—but never quite enough. She still recalls that each time she watched her mother at the grocery store, mentally subtracting items at checkout, her "stomach knotted tighter."

In college, the financial pressure only grew. Every purchase was a battle between need and guilt. She once skipped meals for three days to buy a required textbook, telling her mother that everything was "fine." The taste of ramen noodles became synonymous with sacrifice.

Her mother's decision to be a stay at home mom for Izzy and her siblings had been a point of tension throughout Izzy's life. A college-educated woman with just a few credit hours shy of her master's degree, her mother had chosen to raise her children full-time. The financial sacrifices were clear. Medicaid, food stamps, and HUD housing were not just support but survival.

Izzy's scholarships felt less like triumphs and more like lifelines. Each one was a temporary reprieve from the anxiety that she might not be able to afford another semester. Even the thought of failing a class was suffocating, not just because of academic pressure, but because of what it might cost.

If I fail, does that make every sacrifice she made for nothing? She would ask herself, staring at her bank account. The balance was a glaring reminder of how much Izzy couldn't afford to fail.

Izzy's mind had become a war zone, where her own thoughts turned against her. Every accomplishment was quickly reinterpreted in her brain. It was not proof of her ability, but further evidence that she'd somehow tricked everyone into believing she was competent. That she belonged.

In her world, there were no shades of gray. Every grade was either a triumph or a disaster. This was only intensified when she entered law school. An A-minus in constitutional law felt like proof she wasn't cut out for law school. If she didn't excel perfectly, she felt she was failing entirely. This all-or-nothing mindset was rooted in her upbringing. Her mother's well-intentioned but relentless mantra of "you can't afford to mess up" echoed in her mind during every exam, every presentation, and every job interview. That constantly echoed in her mind. *No room for mistakes, no allowance for learning curves or progress.*

For Izzy, one minor mistake could spiral into a full-blown catastrophe. During a moot court competition, she forgot a case citation and stumbled. The oversight was minor. It was hardly noticed by her peers or judges. But her mind latched onto it and turned it into a nightmare. *If I can't remember one case, I'll fail the bar. If I fail the bar, I'll never get a job. If I can't get a job, everything I've worked for will be worthless.*

By the time the competition ended, she was already planning her apology email to her professor, mentally drafting an explanation for why she wasn't cut out for law. Thankfully, she never wrote it.

Izzy's internal monologues were brutal. Every achievement was either luck, a fluke, or someone else's mistake. When she graduated with honors, her first thought wasn't pride but suspicion. *They probably lowered the standards this year. It doesn't really count.*

Even when her mother framed her diploma—hands trembling slightly as she hung it on the wall—Izzy couldn't look at it without feeling like a fraud. It hung there, evidence she couldn't accept.

The Bar Exam: Am I Strong Enough to Try Again?

Failing the bar exam the first time took her breath away. She was shocked to her core. When she saw the results, Izzy's mind flooded with a single, terrifying question: *Am I strong enough to try again?*

She spent that night in silence, lying on her bed with the lights off, the notification still open on her phone. The shame was suffocating, a weight pressing down until her chest ached. She just kept wondering, *how do I tell my mother?* The thought of her mother's eyes, tired but proud, made her throat tighten.

For weeks, Izzy couldn't bring herself to study again. Every time she opened a textbook, the words seemed to mock her. One of her professor's emails, short and straightforward, finally broke through. "Failure is not proof of inadequacy. Trying again is proof of strength."

Izzy Revisited:

Isabella's story is one of origins. Childhood lessons, racial dynamics, financial struggles, and an ADHD diagnosis intertwined to form a powerful, persistent imposter syndrome. Her story, however, is also a story of defiance. For every voice that told her she wasn't enough, there was another quieter, but just as insistent, voice that reminded her that survival itself was proof of her strength.

I am proud to say that as of this writing, Izzy has passed the bar exam and has been on cloud nine for the last few days. Although her confidence took a blow, it has been greatly restored. And it has grown. She knows that she still has work to do to maintain that resilience, confidence and not to allow herself to get down and stay there.

Her journey to break free from imposter syndrome is ongoing. Marked by small but significant acts of reframing achievements, embracing imperfection, and owning her worth. The fight isn't about erasing self-doubt entirely. She has developed enough self-awareness to learn that is an impossible goal. Maybe she is right; we shall see. Nonetheless, she has triumphed. She has learned to live with it without letting it dictate every decision. Every achievement. Every moment of pride.

The financial hardships that once made every dollar feel like a debt to repay have become a testament to her resilience. Cognitive distortions once twisted every achievement into evidence of fraud. Now they are challenged by tangible proof in her "success journal" and the affirmations she repeats daily. Even the bar exam, despite the initial results, has become an affirmation of her strength and resilience.

I know Izzy quite well and she is a true hustler. Her family's financial struggles created an unshakeable work ethic in her. As hard a worker as she is, pales only to how fierce of an advocate she is for the people and causes that spark her passion. To be clear, the voices of self-doubt are still there. They are much quieter now, but still present. Some days, they are almost silent. Other days, they are deafening. Through every battle, Isabella has learned to remind herself of one truth, her *achievements are real. She has earned her success!*

Chapter 3

The Five Imposter Types

The Many Faces of Imposter Syndrome

Imposter syndrome is a complex psychological pattern that transcends simple self-doubt. It is a deep-seated fear of being exposed as a fraud. This is despite clear evidence of competence and success. For high achievers, this fear is a constant, exhausting presence, transforming success into a source of anxiety rather than validation. The roots of imposter syndrome are often buried in societal pressures, cultural narratives, and early family dynamics that define worth through achievement, perfection, and self-reliance.

Understanding imposter syndrome requires more than acknowledging self-doubt. It demands an exploration of the various ways it manifests. Dr. Valerie Young's research categorizes imposter syndrome into five primary types: the Perfectionist, the Superhero, the Natural Genius, the Soloist, and the Expert.[xvi] Each type represents a distinct strategy for coping with the fear of inadequacy. Each is shaped by unique combinations of upbringing, societal expectations, and personal beliefs about competence.

The challenge is not merely to identify these types but to unravel the societal and psychological narratives that sustain them. By doing so, we can begin to dismantle the false beliefs that keep even the most capable individuals from embracing their achievements fully.

The Five Imposter Types: A Closer Analysis

The Perfectionist — "If I make a mistake, I don't belong here."

For the Perfectionist, success is not an event but a tightrope walk. Any misstep confirms their worst fears of inadequacy. The Perfectionist equates worth with flawlessness. They view even minor errors as proof of incompetence. A lot of us get stuck in this fear of failure that runs so deep, we feel like we can't afford to slip, not even once. So we over-prepare, obsess over every detail, and avoid handing things off. Deep down, we're scared someone else might see the cracks we're trying to hide. It's exhausting, and it's a fast track to burnout.

The roots of perfectionist tendencies are often found in childhood environments where mistakes were met with criticism, rather than guidance. Families that prioritized achievement without balancing it with messages of unconditional support can leave children internalizing the belief that their value is contingent upon perfection. Over time, this belief hardens into a relentless need to control outcomes, which prevents Perfectionists from seeing mistakes as learning opportunities.

The all-or-nothing mindset of the Perfectionist also reflects broader societal messages that equate success with flawlessness. Industries that reward precision—such as law, medicine, and finance—further entrench this belief. They make it more difficult for Perfectionists to see their achievements as sufficient. To overcome this, it is essential to shift from an all-or-nothing approach to a growth mindset that values progress over perfection.

Admittedly, this has been a struggle for me.

My Story, Continued:

Early in my career, I had been assigned to defend a court-appointed client. He had been falsely and egregiously accused of inappropriately touching his two stepchildren. In total, he had thirty-six counts—thirty-six separate accusations. He was not likable. He was loud, scattered in his thinking, and adamant that he knew better than me. Honestly, I wanted to knock him out myself. None of this was helpful to the fact that I was horrified by failing. *If I blew this, he could be going away for life.*

Fast forward, we won. Not guilty on all thirty-six counts. I won on a Rule 29 Motion. Meaning, after the prosecution presented their case, I made an Oral Motion that the case should be dismissed because they did not prove all of the elements (components) of their case. When the judge's gavel banged, it echoed throughout the courtroom. *Did I just win? Did I actually just become a lawyer, finally?*

That elation lasted for a few hours before I got in my own head. *Was that just luck? Was the prosecution just that bad? Did I spend too much time preparing and this should have come to me quicker?*

I couldn't even let myself celebrate. I didn't tell anyone about the win for weeks. And when I finally did, I downplayed it—shrugged, mumbled something about the prosecution falling short. I didn't frame it as a testament to my preparation, my analysis, or my ability to advocate under pressure. I framed it as circumstantial. As luck. Because deep down, I still didn't believe I had done it *right*—not by my impossible standards.

The truth is, even in victory, I felt exposed. I couldn't internalize the moment as competence because I had convinced myself that real lawyers didn't struggle that much. I was embarrassed at how many days, weeks and months that it took me to prepare for that trial. How many times I checked, re-checked, and checked again where I was placing punctuation in briefs, going through my opening arguments, practicing my objections, etc. And since I had labored and obsessed and wrung every ounce of certainty out of the process—I assumed I didn't belong. I couldn't let the win be enough because I hadn't been perfect.

I was so embarrassed I never submitted my bill to the court. *If they saw how much I put into this, they would realize that I had no idea what I was doing.* I flushed $500 down the toilet for fear of being found out as a fraud. As not being perfect.

The Superhero— "I must work harder than everyone else to prove I belong."

The "Superhero" feels like they've got to outwork everybody just to prove they belong. Resting feels like failure. If they can't juggle everything perfectly, they feel flawed. What's really going on within them is a fear that if they ever slow down, people will see through them and realize they're not as competent as they appear.

This mindset doesn't come out of nowhere. It's fed by a culture that glorifies the grind! Hustling nonstop equates to greater value and, presumably, more success. For those from marginalized backgrounds, that pressure is even heavier. When you're constantly battling stereotypes or navigating spaces that doubt your ability, working twice as hard doesn't feel optional. It's a requirement.

Breaking out of the Superhero trap means redefining what makes you worthy. You have to reevaluate your boundaries. Learn to see rest as part of the game plan. Then, recognize that asking for help or delegating isn't a weakness. It is wisdom. Putting a greater value on experiences (such as time with family and friends) and not accolades and/or material possessions helps reposition your thinking. When you stop tying your worth to how exhausted you are, you give yourself permission to work from a place of confidence, not fear.

The Natural Genius— "If I struggle, it means I'm not smart enough."

The Natural Genius equates effort with inadequacy. For this type, the need to try is itself a sign of failure. They believe that true competence should come easy. This mindset is so foul because it convinces so-called "Natural Geniuses" that if something doesn't come easy, it means they're not really cut out for it. Instead of seeing struggle as part of the learning curve, they take it as proof they don't belong. This keeps them from leaning into the very challenges that could help them grow.

This type often emerges in those who were praised for their innate talent rather than effort during childhood. When success is attributed to being naturally gifted rather than to hard work, it creates a fragile self-concept that cannot withstand failure. As adults, Natural Geniuses tend to avoid areas outside their expertise. Subconsciously, they think that trying and failing will expose them as frauds.

To counter this mindset, it is crucial to understand that effort and struggle are vital to mastering your craft. Shifting the focus from effortless achievement to continuous learning can help dismantle the illusion that struggle means you are. You must recognize that expertise is built through persistence, not perfection. Only then will the Natural Geniuses pursue growth without fearing exposure.

Amaka's story helps illustrate this concept more.

The Fall of the Natural Genius: Amaka's Story

Amaka Okoye was always ahead. She enrolled in college at fifteen, not because anyone pushed her, but because it felt natural. She'd always been the one who got it quickly, who read fast, who solved problems without much effort. In high school, she sat beside adults in college classrooms and quietly outpaced them. Being exceptional wasn't something she chased. It was who she was.

And for a long time, it worked.

Born to two Yoruba parents and raised in a faith-centered household outside of Chicago, Amaka grew up with a deep sense of identity. But also, she had a deep sense of pressure. She didn't identify as "Black" in the cultural sense; she was Nigerian. That distinction shaped her early years. It was how she saw herself, how others saw her, and what she believed was expected of her.

As a child, people praised her intelligence more than her effort. "You're so smart," they'd say. "So advanced. So mature." When she got top grades or mastered material faster than her peers, it wasn't framed as the result of discipline or practice. It was seen as evidence of something innate. And Amaka believed it. She wore "smart" like a crown. But what she didn't realize was that the crown came with a trap: if brilliance is who you are, what does it mean if you start to struggle?

The Collapse of Ease

Law school answered that question.

By the time she enrolled, Amaka had already completed a degree in public safety management, interned with the local court, and secured a prestigious clerkship. She entered law school confident and secure in her academic identity. She believed she could outwork anything. And at first, she did.

But law school wasn't like anything she'd experienced. The reading never ended. The grading curve was brutal. And for the first time in her academic life, the rules were unclear. Her confidence began to crack. In her legal writing course, a professor told her that her analysis was strong, but she hadn't spotted enough issues. He gave her a D on her midterm exam.

I thought writing was my strength. I'd always been told that. So when I saw that grade, it didn't just sting, it rewrote my story. I wondered if everyone had been lying to me this whole time. Was I just never that smart to begin with?

That one grade planted doubt. The bar exam cemented it.

Amaka didn't pass.

She was stunned. Not just by the result, but by how deeply it shook her. Her lowest score? The writing section.

It wasn't just disappointing. It felt like a betrayal of everything I thought I was good at.

From the Bench to the Background

The failure had professional consequences. Because she hadn't passed the bar, Amaka was required to step down from her law clerk position with the court. This was a role she had earned through years of diligence and reputation. And now it was being stripped away. In an act of support, the court allowed her to stay on in an administrative capacity. It was a gesture of grace. But to Amaka, it felt like a silent demotion.

> *On paper, it was stable. But inside, I felt like I had been benched. I went from researching cases and helping draft opinions to sitting in the background. I still showed up, still worked hard. But something in me had changed. I felt invisible. Like I was no longer who I said I was.*

As of this writing, Amaka has not retaken the bar.

She hasn't decided whether she will.

When Identity Is Built on Effortless Excellence

Amaka's imposter syndrome didn't begin with law school. It began with brilliance. With being told, over and over, that "she was gifted. She was special. She was meant to lead." When everything came easily, it reinforced the story that she didn't need to try too hard. That she *shouldn't* have to.

Effort suddenly became necessary and failure still followed. Her entire sense of self came undone. This is the defining trait of the Natural Genius imposter type: the belief that *struggle means inadequacy.*

She didn't just fail a test.

She failed a narrative.

> *The people around me still believed in me. The court wanted me to stay. But I didn't believe in myself. I thought, "if I have to work this hard to pass... maybe I was never cut out for this in the first place."*

The tragedy of the Natural Genius isn't in their intelligence, it's in their silence. Because when things stop being easy, they retreat. They don't ask for help. They don't share their struggle. They just internalize their shame. For Amaka, that silence nearly swallowed her confidence.

But over time, she's learning that the ease she once relied on isn't the only way to measure potential. That real brilliance shows up not just when things are smooth, but when they're hard. When you keep going anyway.

She hasn't rewritten her ending yet. However, she's at least started to write a different middle for herself.

The Soloist — "If I ask for help, I will be seen as incompetent."

The Soloist's fear is rooted in the belief that independence equals competence. For them, asking for help is the same as admitting they are a fraud. As a result, they take on excessive workloads, refuse to delegate, and avoid any form of support. This tendency not only leads to burnout but also prevents them from building collaborations, which we know is a tool for success.

The Soloist mindset usually develops in environments that frown upon vulnerability, such as families that equate self-sufficiency with strength or workplaces that penalize mistakes. Over time, the fear of appearing weak morphs into a belief that accepting help will confirm the very incompetence they seek to conceal.

Breaking free from this mindset requires redefining that need to be unhealthily independent. True competence is not about doing everything alone but about knowing when to seek support. They must embrace that collaboration can be a strategic advantage rather than a sign of weakness. In doing so, the Soloist can now begin to see partnering with others or delegating tasks as signs of leadership, not liabilities.

The Expert—"I need more credentials before I can be considered successful."

The Expert sees knowledge and credentials as the ultimate proof of their competence. For this type, no amount of experience ever feels sufficient. There is always more to learn. This endless pursuit of qualifications is not about growth but about managing the fear of being exposed as unqualified.

The Expert mindset is often reinforced by professional environments that prioritize credentials over capability. In fields where expertise is synonymous with authority, the pressure to accumulate certifications and degrees becomes a defensive strategy against being found out.

To overcome the Expert mindset, it is essential to differentiate between the pursuit of knowledge for growth and the pursuit of knowledge to conceal fear. Recognizing that true expertise is not about knowing everything but about continuous learning can help shift the focus from proving competence to embracing it. Confidence grows not from the accumulation of credentials but from the ability to apply what you have learned.

The Reluctant Expert: Chasing Credentials to Prove His Worth

Darius Vaughn spent his life believing that success required *just one more credential.* Raised in Charlotte, North Carolina, he was a high-achiever who never felt truly seen. As a child he was heavy set and bullied, so he did not fit in easily. As he matured, he grew, leaned out and started to receive attention and became popular. Nonetheless, he didn't become confident. This was exacerbated by the fact that although he excelled in school, he was overlooked by teachers. He downplayed his own intelligence. He feared that any mistake would expose him as unworthy.

At Morehouse College, his perfectionism deepened. He overprepared, joined multiple organizations, and pushed himself relentlessly. He remained convinced that his accomplishments were never enough. Though he eventually earned a finance degree, he pivoted to cybersecurity, seeking stability. Even as he mastered new skills, he doubted his expertise. He continued to collect certifications in his endless quest for validation.

45

When invited to present a high-profile software project that had saved his company millions, imposter syndrome took hold. Facing a room of senior executives, he convinced himself they would see through him. When an older colleague undermined him mid-presentation, he shrank back, deferring to those who had quietly relied on his expertise all along.

Darius' Epiphany:

That moment hit hard, but not in the way he expected. Being publicly undermined didn't confirm his worst fears. It actually had the unintended benefit of teaching him that more credentials could protect him from self-doubt. The real problem wasn't his knowledge. It was his belief that he needed external validation to prove it. For the first time, he realized he'd been working to outrun a feeling, not a fact.

He started unpacking that mindset. He talked more with his mentors. He reflected on his journey, and slowly let go of the idea that he had to earn his seat every single day. Now, as a cybersecurity professional and mentor to young Black IT specialists, Darius teaches that success isn't about having every credential. It is about owning what you already know, speaking up when it counts, and refusing to shrink to make others comfortable. He leads with confidence, not perfectionism—and that has made all the difference.

Reclaiming Authentic Confidence: You Were Never the Fraud

The five imposter types are not inherent flaws. They are survival strategies shaped by societal messages that equate worth with achievement, independence, and flawlessness. Breaking free from these patterns begins with challenging the distorted beliefs that sustain them.

Confidence is not the absence of self-doubt, but the ability to move forward despite it. Reclaiming authentic confidence involves recognizing that self-doubt is a product of unrealistic standards and false narratives about your competence. Embrace your imperfection. Seek the support without feeling guilty or incompetent. Value your progress over perfection. Then it becomes possible for you to move from just surviving to being vastly more self-assured.

Imposter syndrome is not about your capabilities. Imposter syndrome is a reflection of the experiences, trauma and conditioning that has shaped your beliefs about your capabilities. Recognizing this distinction is the first step toward dismantling the false narratives that keep you from embracing your right to lead, contribute, and belong.

Chapter 4

Why Imposter Syndrome Hits Harder for Some

Introduction: How Structural Barriers Shape Feelings of Not Belonging

For many professionals, imposter syndrome is more than just an internal battle with self-doubt. It is heightened by a world that consistently marginalizes them. While traditional narratives suggest that imposter syndrome is an individual issue, rooted in personal insecurities, the reality is far more complex.

Marginalized professionals—including people of color, women, LGBTQIA+ individuals, first-generation graduates, neurodivergent professionals, and those from lower-income backgrounds—do not experience imposter syndrome just because of their internal self-doubt. The barriers that exist within education, careers, and opportunities overall place a great weight around their necks. These barriers manifest as implicit biases in hiring and promotions, pay disparities, the constant need to prove oneself, and the lack of diverse representation in leadership roles. 'Implicit bias refers to the attitudes or stereotypes that affect our understanding, actions, and decisions in an unconscious manner. These biases are activated involuntarily, without awareness or intentional control, and can influence behavior even when individuals consciously reject prejudiced attitudes."[xvii]

Imposter syndrome does not develop in a vacuum. It is not exclusively an internal struggle for some. It is a rational response to systemic inequities that continually remind them that they do not belong - or are not welcome. When workplaces and institutions create environments where only a select few feel truly welcome, it is no surprise that so many talented individuals struggle with self-doubt. Overcoming imposter syndrome, then, is not just about shifting your mindset. It is about dismantling the systems that perpetuate it.

The Role of Identity and Systemic Barriers

Professional spaces are often built around unspoken norms that center whiteness, masculinity, and heterosexuality. These norms determine what leadership looks like, how competence is evaluated, and who gets the benefit of the doubt. Those who do not naturally fit into these expectations often find themselves having to work twice as hard, downplay aspects of their identity, or constantly prove their value.

One of the more subtle but draining ways imposter syndrome shows up is through code switching. For many professionals of color and LGBTQIA+ individuals, thriving at work often means adjusting how they talk, dress, or carry themselves to align with dominant workplace norms. It becomes a performance that might gain you access to the room, but at the cost of feeling fully seen. *What does it mean when success requires leaving parts of yourself at the door?* That repeated message that your natural way of being isn't "professional enough" can erode your confidence over time. It reinforces the lie that authenticity is a risk and that who you are isn't enough.[xviii]

Beyond cultural expectations, marginalized professionals also face harsher scrutiny. A simple mistake can reinforce stereotypes about incompetence. Meanwhile, others are allowed to fail and recover without consequence. Women, for example, are often penalized for being too assertive while simultaneously being overlooked if they are too accommodating. Professionals of color are frequently held to higher standards yet receive less recognition for their work. These realities make imposter syndrome more than just an internal fear. It becomes evidence of how bias can determine who has their opportunities limited or expanded.

People of Color and Imposter Syndrome: The Burden of Proof

For people of color—including Black, Indigenous, Latino/Latina/Latinx individuals—imposter syndrome is profoundly shaped by the need to prove competence beyond a reasonable doubt. The pressure to be "twice as good" is not just a motivational saying. I do not know a single Black person who has never said that to themselves. It becomes a survival strategy because we know that mistakes are often seen as proof of unfitness rather than opportunities for growth.

Implicit biases in hiring, performance evaluations, and promotions ensure that people of color are scrutinized more closely, praised less frequently, and advanced more slowly than their white counterparts. This creates a continuous, and unintended, need to overcompensate. We work longer hours, accept more tasks, and avoid risks that might expose any perceived incompetence.

Code-switching further compounds this burden. Continuously monitoring speech, behavior, and appearance to conform to predominantly white professional norms is mentally exhausting. It reinforces the belief that being ourselves can be a liability. Success is only possible by hiding aspects of our true identity. This form of imposter syndrome is not about internal doubt; it is about navigating a world that explicitly tells you that who you are is not enough.

Women and Imposter Syndrome: The Double Bind

Being a woman in leadership already comes with a double bind.[xix] You're expected to be competent, but also warm and agreeable. Push too hard and you're labeled aggressive. Show too much empathy and you're dismissed as weak. It's a tightrope that's as exhausting as it is unfair.

Now add race to that equation, and the bind tightens. Vice President Kamala Harris is a textbook example. She was more than qualified by any traditional measure—former Senator, Attorney General of California, Howard University grad, HBCU and Divine Nine legacy. But for many Americans, that wasn't enough. Or rather, it was too much. The fact that she was a Black woman with ambition, intellect, and power made her polarizing before she even opened her mouth. The media on both sides made this clear. Suddenly, being a stepmother was held against her. Her background as a prosecutor was twisted into a liability. And the absence of a narrowly defined "Black agenda" became a weapon, as if she was supposed to carry the full weight of America's racial healing on her shoulders alone.

That's the double bind in action. Anything you do can and will be used against you. And it's not just frustrating; it's career-defining. Women who self-promote get labeled arrogant. Women who stay humble get ignored. Many end up over-preparing, refusing to delegate, and grinding themselves down just to be seen as "enough." The fear of confirming stereotypes about women's capability becomes so strong that it fuels perfectionism and burnout.[xx] Men have a level of grace that allows us to fail without lasting damage. Well, some of us. However, women, especially women of color, know that even a small misstep can cost them everything.

This isn't just imposter syndrome born in the mind. It's reinforced by how the world responds to women when they dare to lead.[xxi]

Lauren Carter's Imposter Syndrome and the Double Bind of Professional Women: A Lifetime of Undervaluing Herself

Lauren Carter's academic and professional journey has been defined by a consistent pattern of downplaying her achievements and failing to advocate for herself. She excelled academically from a young age, attending competitive schools and proving herself in rigorous environments. Yet, despite her intelligence and capability, she rarely took ownership of her success. Instead, she attributed her accomplishments to luck, timing, or external factors rather than recognizing her own talent and effort.

This mindset carried over into law school. Even after passing the bar exam on her first attempt, she struggled to secure an attorney position. Rather than seeing herself as an asset to potential employers, she doubted whether she belonged in the legal field at all. With no immediate job offers, she opened her own practice. She did not do it because she was that confident in herself. She did it out of a perceived necessity. She handled cases across multiple legal areas, constantly learning and adapting, but without mentorship or structured support, she struggled to build long-term professional security. Instead of viewing this experience as proof of her resilience and skill, she saw it as further evidence that she was figuring things out rather than actually succeeding.

Choosing Security Over Ambition

As financial pressures mounted, Lauren took a temporary position in bankruptcy law, intending to work there only briefly before returning to practice as an attorney. That temporary job turned into fifteen years. During that time, she remained in the same role, never seeking promotions or advocating for salary increases. Her employers never questioned why she stayed in the same position, and she never pushed for advancement.

Even when she learned that a less-experienced colleague was earning significantly more, she did not raise the issue or request a salary adjustment. Instead, she blamed herself for not negotiating in the beginning. This reinforced her cycle of self-doubt and inaction. When she finally decided to leave the job, she accepted the first salary offer from her new employer without negotiation. To be clear, she knew it still did not reflect her worth. She accepted it simply because it was more than she "had been making before."

This pattern highlights the professional cost of imposter syndrome. Despite being fully qualified, Lauren consistently relegated herself to roles beneath her abilities and accepted whatever was given to her, rather than actively seeking what she deserved.

The Double Bind: Assertiveness vs. Likability

Lauren's experience mirrors the double bind that many professional women face. They must be competent but not intimidating, confident but not arrogant.

Throughout her career, she hesitated to assert herself out of fear of being perceived as ungrateful or demanding. If she spoke up too much, would she be seen as aggressive? If she didn't, would she be overlooked? This tension kept her in a frustrating cycle of wanting more responsibility but hesitating to demand it.

At one point, when a senior colleague left her firm, leadership reassigned her responsibilities. But not to Lauren. Despite being told in prior evaluations that she was ready for a more senior role, she was passed over without explanation. Rather than asking why or pushing for the leadership role she had earned, she convinced herself that perhaps she wasn't quite ready after all.

This reluctance to self-advocate is a tell-tell sign of imposter syndrome. When women hesitate to highlight their own achievements, they risk being perceived as passive or unambitious. Thereby reinforcing the very barriers that keep them from advancing.

Checking in with Lauren Carter:

Today, Lauren is a law librarian at a prestigious firm and has set a five-year goal to move into a senior leadership role. However, she still wrestles with the same internal questions. *How does she stand out? Is she truly ready? Will she ever feel fully qualified?*

Though she is making small steps toward asserting herself and taking ownership of her expertise, it remains a challenge. Years of internalizing self-doubt have made it difficult for her to break free from the tendency to wait for opportunities rather than demand them.

Her story is a powerful example of how women's imposter syndrome is not just about self-doubt. It is shaped by workplace expectations, biases, and the constant balancing act of ambition versus likability. When self-doubt intersects with these structural challenges, even the most capable and qualified women can end up settling for less than they deserve—not because they lack ability, but because they hesitate to claim their space.

LGBTQIA+ Professionals: The Dilemma of Authenticity

For LGBTQIA+ professionals, imposter syndrome is compounded by the fear of discrimination in heteronormative workplaces. The choice to conceal or reveal one's identity becomes a continuous calculation of risks. Hiding your true self makes it harder to fully embrace your achievements. It reinforces the idea that your success is fragile and might not last. However, openness brings its own challenges—exposing LGBTQIA+ professionals to tokenism,[xxii] microaggressions, and scrutiny that their cisgender,[xxiii] heterosexual colleagues rarely encounter.

The scarcity of openly LGBTQIA+ leaders in senior positions intensifies this isolation. According to a 2021 McKinsey report, LGBTQ+ women and transgender employees often feel isolated in the workplace. This isolation leads to a more negative experience and affects their motivation to pursue leadership roles.[xxiv] This lack of representation can contribute to a sense of invisibility and marginalization. It sends an implicit message that leadership is incompatible with queerness. It reinforces the fear that their presence is contingent on silence and assimilation rather than competence and authenticity.

Navigating this landscape often requires adopting perfectionist behaviors. They must avoid making mistakes at all costs, over prepare for every task, and refuse to seek help. The nonstop grind drains energy, reinforces imposter feelings, and creates the illusion that any success is just a short-lived stroke of luck.

This was the experience of Jonathan Pierce, an openly gay Black man who spent years excelling in workplaces that were eager to benefit from his expertise but reluctant to recognize his leadership.

The Silent Struggle: Jonathan Pierce's Experience with Being Overlooked

Jonathan Pierce never lacked talent or ambition, yet time and again, he found himself fighting to be fully acknowledged.

Raised in Jackson, Mississippi, Jonathan spent much of his life adapting to new environments. As a child, he moved from a predominantly Black neighborhood to a mostly white school district. He quickly learned that his presence was tolerated, but not necessarily welcomed. His teachers often underestimated him. They assumed he needed remedial assistance instead of recognizing that he was simply navigating an environment where he was one of the few Black students. He was learning unspoken social rules that others took for granted.

His imposter syndrome didn't begin because he doubted himself. It began because, at every turn, he was given subtle and overt messages that he was not meant to be in these spaces.

After high school, he initially enrolled in a local community college before enlisting in the military under "Don't Ask, Don't Tell." His service during Operation Iraqi

Freedom brought discipline and resilience, but it also reinforced the reality that he needed to hide his gay identity for survival in the military.

After his military service, Jonathan pursued a degree in social work and public health, quickly rising in nonprofit leadership. His expertise was undeniable. He managed teams, secured funding, and developed programs that helped underserved communities gain access to healthcare. Yet, time and again, he found that his voice was only acknowledged when it was convenient.

At one nonprofit, he led an HIV prevention initiative focused on Black men. Though he was the one who had designed the program, built relationships with the community, and understood its needs, his white colleagues often dismissed his ideas. That is, until they needed him to speak on behalf of the Black community. He was included when it benefited them but excluded from leadership decisions that shaped the program.

Jonathan had long internalized that perfection was a requirement, not an option. He avoided mistakes at all costs, overprepared for every presentation, and worked twice as hard to ensure there was no room for criticism. He hesitated to ask for help, fearing it would be seen as incompetence rather than collaboration. Over time, the pressure to overperform became overwhelming. This led to both burnout and a stronger belief that he didn't truly belong. His achievements, no matter how significant, never felt like solid ground. They were only a temporary reprieve before he had to prove himself all over again.

The peak of his imposter syndrome came when he was promoted to interim executive director of a struggling organization. Under his leadership, he secured major funding, restructured operations, and stabilized programs. Yet, when the time came to make his role permanent, the board hesitated. His qualifications were not the issue. His ability to lead had already been proven. He felt that the hesitation came from the discomfort of placing a young, openly gay Black man in charge of an organization that had historically been led by straight white executives.

Jonathan was left with a painful, yet empowering realization. His imposter syndrome was not rooted in his own doubts, but in the reluctance of others to fully recognize him. He had done everything right, yet the pathway to advancement remained obstructed. Eventually, he stepped away. He needed to find a work community that saw and heard him, not just tokenized him when it was convenient to do so.

Jonathan Pierce Revisited:

Johnathan is now a vice president at another organization. He is still often the only Black leader in executive spaces. But he no longer waits for permission to be heard. Ironically, Jonathan was always comfortable in his identity as a Black, openly gay man. He did not see these traits as separate from who he was. They were all parts of his identity. His imposter syndrome did not stem from his race or sexuality. He felt unseen and unheard, period.

For him, why he was invisible was a secondary concern. Whether it was because he was Black, gay or Black and gay was insignificant to him. He just wanted to be recognized as the effective leader that he was. The reality is that people may have just been intimidated by him because he was a young, educated professional who was willing to share his opinion, especially when he saw inefficient processes and procedures. In a system that rewards deference over disruption, his presence was unsettling.

Reclaiming Authenticity and Redefining Success

Overcoming imposter syndrome for marginalized groups requires redefining success. It must include authenticity, impact, and alignment with personal values rather than perfection or assimilation. It means recognizing that self-doubt is often a rational response to external biases rather than proof of incompetence.

Building networks with others who share similar experiences can also counteract the isolation that fuels imposter syndrome. Sponsors who actively advocate for the advancement of marginalized professionals—rather than just providing mentorship—are crucial for opening those exclusionary doors.

Conclusion: Challenging Systems, Reclaiming Confidence

Imposter syndrome is not always the result of an internal struggle. It can be the result of systemic inequities that must be challenged. Recognizing the external factors that perpetuate self-doubt is essential for reclaiming confidence and redefining what it means to belong. By distinguishing self-doubt from systemic barriers, seeking sponsors who can advocate for us, and reframing success on our own terms, we can begin to silence the inner critic that questions our right to lead, succeed, and thrive.

In doing so, we transform imposter syndrome from a burden into a catalyst for change, for ourselves and for the systems that have made us feel unwelcome.

Overcoming imposter syndrome is not about learning to be more confident in a broken system. It is about challenging the system itself. By advocating for equity in hiring, leadership opportunities, and workplace culture, we can move towards a reality where belonging is not something we have to fight for, but something that is freely given.

Success should not require erasure. It should not require proving oneself over and over again just to be seen. It is time to redefine success on our own terms.

PART II

REWIRING YOUR MINDSET

Chapter 5

The Science Behind Imposter Syndrome:

Introduction: Imposter Syndrome as a Hardwired Brain Response

I am not a neuroscientist or a psychologist. I had to deeply research this chapter because I understand that many readers may want to know the science behind why they feel the way they do. For those who value a deeper understanding of the brain's role in imposter syndrome, this chapter explores the neurological, psychological, and cognitive factors that drive self-doubt. By demystifying the science, my goal is to help you develop more effective habits, routines, and strategies to navigate it in your own life.

Imposter syndrome is often seen as a sign of insecurity or a lack of confidence. At its core, it is a deeply ingrained neurological and psychological response. It's not just an emotional reaction. It is how our brains are wired to respond to perceived risk, social evaluation, and uncertainty.

The human brain is inherently wired to prioritize survival, making it more sensitive to threats—both physical and social—than to positive experiences like success or praise. This heightened vigilance is rooted in our evolutionary history, where detecting and responding to threats was crucial for survival. Neuroscientific research indicates that the brain's threat response systems are more readily activated and have a stronger impact on behavior than reward systems. For instance, the amygdala plays a central role in processing threats, triggering rapid responses to perceived dangers, while reward processing involves different neural circuits that are less immediately reactive.[xxv]

For a lot of high achievers, self-doubt isn't about falling short. It is about survival. It's something they picked up from living in a world that, in subtle and not-so-subtle ways, kept telling them they didn't belong. Layer that with the weight of mental health (whether it runs in your family, comes from your environment, or both) and the pressure multiplies. That's when you realize imposter syndrome isn't always something you developed as an adult. For many of us, it started way earlier, quietly absorbed through experiences long before we even had the language to name it.

How the Brain Processes Self-Doubt

At its core, the brain is wired for survival, not success. That means it's naturally inclined to avoid risk and steer clear of uncertainty.[xxvi] When imposter syndrome kicks in, two key brain regions take center stage: the amygdala, which sets off the "fear alarm,"[xxvii] and the prefrontal cortex, which is supposed to handle logic, reasoning, and decision-making. But here's the cruel irony. When that fear gets loud, it drowns out the rational part of the brain. So something as routine as speaking up in a meeting or receiving critical feedback can feel like a full-blown threat, not just a bump in the road. This isn't just a mindset issue. It's how our brains are wired when fear overrides reason.[xxviii]

The Amygdala: The Brain's Fear Center

The amygdala is a small, almond-shaped structure nestled deep within the brain's limbic system. Its primary role is to process emotions, especially fear.[xxix] The amygdala will then trigger the body's fight-or-flight response when it perceives a threat.[xxx] In our evolution, this was a lifesaving function. Early humans could then react quickly to predators or danger.[xxxi] But in today's world, the amygdala's fear response often gets activated in situations that are not life-threatening but still feel high-stakes. Activities such as giving a presentation, applying for a promotion or stepping into a leadership role can all trigger this response.[xxxii]

Understanding that these responses are driven by a part of the brain that is hardwired for survival can help you approach your self-doubt with more compassion and less judgment. It also suggests that strategies to calm the amygdala—such as deep breathing, mindfulness, or grounding exercises—can be effective in managing imposter syndrome.[xxxiii]

The Prefrontal Cortex: The Brain's Logic Center

Unlike the amygdala, which runs on emotion and instinct, the prefrontal cortex (PFC) is the more level-headed part of your brain. This is where logic, decision-making, and self-control live.[xxxiv] When things are calm, the PFC helps talk the amygdala down, putting fear into perspective and reminding you of past wins and real evidence that you're capable.[xxxv]

But chronic stress, which is pervasive in folks dealing with imposter syndrome, throws that balance off. Under pressure, the PFC doesn't fully function. Its ability to calm your emotions and think rationally gets hijacked,[xxxvi] leaving you more vulnerable to irrational fear and less able to talk yourself off the ledge with facts.

I am sure that you have had moments where you knew, intellectually, that you were prepared. Think of your last job interview. You did your homework, knew the right answers to give and the perfect questions to ask. You had the credentials and the experience. You knew you would nail the interview.

"But wait, am I qualified for this job," you asked yourself. *Did I prepare enough? Will they learn about that "C" I got in 8th grade science?* You start hearing "Lose Yourself" by Eminem echoing in your head:

> "His palms are sweaty, knees weak, arms are heavy
> There's vomit on his sweater already: Mom's spaghetti
> He's nervous, but on the surface he looks calm and ready

To drop bombs, but he keeps on forgetting
What he wrote down, the whole crowd goes so loud
He opens his mouth, but the words won't come out
He's choking, how? Everybody's joking now..."[xxxvii]

Your mind and body aren't connected. The memo was not circulated to your body that you were ready. The fear still came. Your voice still shook. That disconnect was your amygdala and PFC playing tug-of-war in real time.

Of course, knowing how your brain works is only part of the story. For many of us, imposter syndrome isn't just about biology. It is also about our biography. Our story. The fear isn't always rooted in what's happening right now. Sometimes it's a lingering shadow from thoughts and/or experiences long gone and forgotten. From growing up around instability. From caretakers who were inconsistent or emotionally unavailable. From early trauma that rewired how your nervous system responds to stress, long before you ever knew what "resilience" meant.[xxxviii]

This is why the praise doesn't always stick. Why even when others see your brilliance, you still second-guess it. Your nervous system is scanning for danger, not applause.

The science matters, but so does the story. To unpack the power imposter syndrome can have over us, we can't just look at what the brain is doing. We have to ask where the fear learned to speak so loudly in the first place.

My Story, Continued: When the Inner Critic Is Inherited

For many of us, imposter syndrome is entangled with generational patterns, family dynamics, and a long history of emotional survival. It's not just a matter of "feeling insecure," it's about being wired for vigilance, shaped by pain, and conditioned by experience.

I've always feared that my own mind might betray me.

Both my mother and my grandmother lived with diagnosed mental illnesses. I grew up in the shadow of those diagnoses, never fully sure what might be lurking in my own DNA. As a child, I watched my mother cycle through manic episodes, hospitalizations, and periods of intense unpredictability. As I got older, I tried to make sense of it, tried to stay strong, tried to stay functional.

But trauma has a way of shaping your expectations. It taught me to be alert at all times, to prepare for chaos, to equate love with caretaking and crisis management.

Then came the United States Marine Corps. More structure, more firepower, more discipline, but also more trauma. As the saying goes, "when I returned to civilian life, I brought something back with me." It lived in me. In my temper. In my inability to sleep. In my sudden shifts from calm to anger. I was functioning. I was performing. I was succeeding on paper. But underneath that? I did not understand who I was. My residual survival instincts stayed that much more heightened. Like some of you reading this now, I cannot sit with my back to an open door or window. I do not walk into a room without scanning it, instinctively, looking for how many exits are there and where they are. In some social settings I cannot relax. I stay alert. That used to cause me to drink too much to try to relax. To try and live in the moment.

When I started law school, I thought things would change. But, changing scenery does not change you, or so I learned. In my first year, I made a decision I had long dreamed of. I would help my mother regain some independence. A classmate and I moved her into her own apartment. I wanted her to have something stable. Something she could call her own. This is what she wanted. I thought she was ready and so did she.

Wrong.

That night, she had a manic episode. She was hospitalized, and she never lived on her own again.

For the next six years, my mother moved between hospitals, my home, residential facilities, and group homes. While I was studying for torts and preparing for oral arguments, I was also fielding emergency phone calls, managing medication plans, and wondering if I was doing enough. Would anything ever be enough?

She ultimately passed away from what they called "failure to thrive." In simple terms, it means her body just stopped fighting. It's a term often used when there's no single cause, just a mix of things—physical, emotional, maybe even spiritual—that slowly wears a person down.

And through it all—law school, the Ohio Bar Exam, launching my legal career, getting hired (and released) from my first firm, and pledging Omega Psi Phi Fraternity,

Inc.—I carried a deep, quiet fear, *what if I'm next? What if I'm broken too?*

Eventually, I stopped dodging those inner questions and sought some answers. I got diagnosed. To be clear, it was almost a decade after she died. After years of unsuccessful therapy and a host of bad decisions, I found the strength to get answers. The labels came—anger management issues, anxiety, PTSD, stress disorder—but oddly, so did relief. It gave shape to what I had been carrying. It offered language for what had always felt like a private war inside my head. *I am a hot mess, but, there is an explanation and some avenue forward.*

I got help. I revisited therapy, committed to it and did the work. I returned to my previous therapist who understood both my trauma and my ambition. Some conversations were more open and honest. Some I probably still lie to myself about. But again, I am a work in progress. Eventually, I even found a medication plan that worked. I started to feel I was okay. Not perfect. Not cured. But, at least, okay.

This is why the neuroscience of imposter syndrome matters. Because sometimes, what we think is a personal flaw is really a hardwired survival response.

My brain was trained to expect threats. My nervous system was calibrated for chaos. I grew up in an environment where violence was not an anomaly. It was a backdrop. Street fights, sirens, the constant awareness that anything could pop off at any moment. That kind of upbringing doesn't just toughen you. It conditions you. It teaches your body to stay on alert, your emotions to stay guarded, and your trust to stay locked behind a thick wall of self-preservation.

So of course, walking into a courtroom or standing before City Council would feel like a test I wasn't ready for.

Even when I was.

Because my body didn't know the difference between real danger and perceived danger, it didn't matter how much I'd prepared. If the room felt like judgment, my nervous system braced for impact.

That's the cruel twist of imposter syndrome when it's rooted in trauma. You can be more qualified than everyone in the room and still feel like the most expendable person in that same room.

Situational Imposter Syndrome: When Context Triggers Self-Doubt

Imposter syndrome isn't always something you carry around all the time. Sometimes, it shows up in specific situations. It can sneak in when you're stepping into a new role, taking on more responsibility, or entering an environment that feels unfamiliar or high-stakes. In these moments, it's not necessarily about trauma, mental health, or deep-rooted self-esteem issues. Sometimes it's just your brain doing what it's wired to do. It is reacting to uncertainty like it's a threat.

Think about someone who's been thriving in a hands-on, technical role and suddenly gets promoted into leadership. The job changes. The spotlight gets brighter. Expectations shift. Even if their skills haven't changed, their brain might kick into fear mode. Now here comes the self-doubt, anxiety, and second-guessing.

This kind of situational imposter syndrome is also common when people enter elite spaces, switch careers, or find themselves as the only one in the room who looks, talks, or thinks like they do. Without a sense of psychological safety, the brain's alarm system goes off, and confidence takes a hit, even when the competence is rock solid.[xxxix]

Renee Wallace knows this experience intimately.

A Life of Shifting: How Renee Wallace Learned to Lead Despite the Doubt

Renee Wallace, a high-performing executive, began her career training senior-level managers at a national insurance firm based in Chicago Renee often found herself as the only Black woman, and frequently the youngest person, in the room. On paper, she was accomplished, confident, and well-prepared. But inside, her nervous system was doing something entirely different. It was constantly scanning for threats.

Long before boardrooms and policy meetings, Renee had learned to navigate her identity through code-switching. She grew up between two very different environments. In North Hartford, the distinctions between race and class were highly visible. In the rural outskirts, being visibly Black meant she had to shrink herself just to feel safe. As a child, she often felt like an outsider. When her mother had a religious conversion, another layer of separation emerged. Renee was pulled from classroom celebrations, discouraged from participating in "worldly" activities, and told that dorm life would lead her away from God.

It wasn't just her environment that shaped her, it was the subtle but persistent message: *You don't fully belong anywhere. Be careful how you show up.*

When she later stepped into corporate spaces—armed with credentials, preparation, and poise—her inner critic was still screaming loudly at her. It was a conditioned defense. Her amygdala wasn't simply reacting to pressure, it was responding to years of coded warnings. And her prefrontal cortex, the brain's logic center, had to fight uphill to override those internal alarms.

Despite numerous promotions and accolades, Renee found herself obsessively rehearsing presentations the night before. She double-checked her language, her appearance, her tone. Not because she doubted her knowledge, but because she *knew* what the consequences of being misunderstood or misjudged could be.

She calls it "role-shifting fatigue". Role-shifting fatigue is that mental and emotional exhaustion that sets in when you're constantly adjusting who you are to fit into spaces where your identity feels spotlighted but not fully supported.[xl] It's a form of situational imposter syndrome that shows up when you're visible, but not safe. It didn't happen in every room. But in the wrong room, it could still paralyze her.

Even now, as a highly educated, highly accomplished professional—serving on nonprofit boards, mentoring young women, and helping design wellness spaces for Black medical professionals—Renee sometimes finds herself second-guessing in the moments where she's most qualified.

She recalls a board meeting where she silently withheld insight, even though the issue being discussed fell directly within her wheelhouse.

"I kept wondering, *Will I say it the right way? Will they assume I'm being emotional or inexperienced?*" she thought. Her old brain programming just kicked back in.

That's what makes situational imposter syndrome so distinct. It's not about incompetence. Stressful environments evoke past fears and reawaken internal defense systems, sometimes louder than ever before.

Renee's healing comes through awareness and action. She names the feeling. She breathes through the response. She grounds herself in evidence. She leans on her faith. She speaks anyway.

She's not waiting for the fear to go away. She owns her authority over it.

And that's the key lesson. Situational imposter syndrome doesn't mean you're in the wrong place. Often, it's a sign that you're stretching and growing into a new version of yourself. And while the fear may still rise, it doesn't have to lead.

Renee's story reminds us that the presence of self-doubt is not proof that we don't belong. It's proof that we're human. We are walking into rooms our ancestors couldn't even dream of. Let your voice shake, let your palms sweat, but walk boldly into that room anyway.

Competing Perspectives on Imposter Syndrome

While the cognitive and neurological explanations of imposter syndrome are compelling, they are not the only perspectives. Several competing theories offer valuable insights into why imposter syndrome occurs and how it can be managed. Understanding these perspectives can provide a more nuanced view of imposter syndrome and offer additional pathways for overcoming it.

Sociocultural Theory: The Impact of Systemic Inequality

What if imposter syndrome isn't a personal flaw at all? Sociocultural theory says it might actually be a rational reaction to the systems we're navigating.[xli] When you're a person of color, a woman, or identify as LGBTQIA+, you're not doubting yourself because you lack confidence. The doubt is born from the spaces you move through constantly, and often loudly, signaling that you don't belong there.[xlii]

From this angle, imposter syndrome isn't just insecurity. It's self-protection. A way of staying mentally alert in spaces that were never built with you in mind.[xliii] If you rarely see someone who looks like you in leadership, it's not surprising that some part of you questions whether you should be there. Even when all the evidence shows you're more than qualified.[xliv]

So the fix isn't just about telling yourself you're good enough. It's about changing the systems that keep sending the message you're not. That means more diverse leadership, fairer feedback, and accountability for bias, spoken or unspoken.[xlv] To be clear, I am not saying that that is easily obtained, but that is a discussion for an entirely different day.

Attachment Theory: The Role of Early Relationships

Attachment theory, first introduced by psychologist John Bowlby, basically says that the way we connect with our earliest caregivers shapes how we see ourselves and how we show up in the world.[xlvi] When we grow up with caregivers who are consistent, supportive, and emotionally available, we tend to develop a solid sense of self-worth. But when that support is inconsistent—when love feels tied to achievement, behavior, or perfection—we often carry that uncertainty into adulthood.[xlvii]

If you learned early on that approval had to be earned, not given, you might still feel like you have to constantly prove yourself to be accepted. That mindset leads to overworking, chasing perfection, and living in fear that people will eventually figure out you're not as capable as they think.[xlviii]

Looking at imposter syndrome through attachment theory isn't just about understanding the past. It is about healing from it. It means learning how to offer yourself the kind of support you may not have received early on. It means building relationships, both personal and professional, where you feel seen, valued, and safe enough to be your full self. Without always having to perform.[xlix]

Evolutionary Psychology: Imposter Syndrome as an Adaptive Mechanism

What if a little self-doubt is actually good for us? According to the evolutionary psychology theory, imposter syndrome, at least in small doses, might be more than just a mental hurdle. It might actually be an adaptive trait that helped our ancestors survive.[l]

Think about it. In environments where the stakes were high and the risks were real, unchecked overconfidence could get you killed. Literally killed. A healthy dose of self-questioning forced early humans to double-check their surroundings, prepare more thoroughly, and think twice before stepping into danger. Remember what I said about sitting with my back to the door or scanning for exits when walking into a room? Survival instincts.

That same wiring, albeit different circumstances, still shows up today. Rehearsing for a presentation ten times, triple-checking my work, or staying up late fine-tuning a project is still a form of survival. Career survival. In moderation, that's not dysfunction, that's vigilance.[li] That is being professional and doing my due-diligence.

I've seen evolutionary psychology play out in my own life. That anxiety I spoke of regarding a job interview, that was my personal experience. Some of my best performances have come after moments of self-doubt. It was not because I believed I wasn't capable, but because I knew I couldn't afford to wing it. After I pulled myself together, I nailed the interview and got that job. That anxiety made me sharper. More prepared. Hungrier to prove myself right—even when a voice inside was whispering I might be wrong.

The problem isn't the self-doubt itself. It is when it refuses to turn off. When it shifts from motivation to paralysis. When no amount of preparation feels like enough. That's when something that was once adaptive becomes a roadblock. A hurdle you can't overcome. A voice that doesn't just push you to do better; it convinces you you're not good enough, no matter what you do.

So maybe the goal isn't to silence imposter syndrome completely. Maybe it's to learn how to manage it. To keep the part that keeps us humble, focused, and prepared, but let go of the part that keeps us stuck, small, and afraid.

Intersectionality Theory: The Amplification of Imposter Syndrome

Intersectionality isn't just a buzzword, it's a lens that helps us see the full picture. Coined by legal scholar Kimberlé Crenshaw, intersectionality theory was developed to explain how systems of oppression don't show up in neat little boxes.[lii] You can't slice someone's identity into just race *or* gender *or* class and expect to understand their experience. That's not how the real world works.

Crenshaw introduced the concept to highlight how Black women, for example, face overlapping forms of discrimination. They do not endure racism *or* sexism, but both at once. They manifest in ways that are unique and often invisible when we look at only one category at a time. It's the difference between asking, "*What's it like to be a woman here?*" and "*What's it like to be a Black woman over there?*" The answers aren't interchangeable.

That, unfortunately, tracks. I know I have been in spaces where being a Black man meant I had to prove I belonged. In those same rooms, I've seen Black women fighting this two-pronged battle. You realize quickly that privilege and oppression aren't one-size-fits-all. They layer. They collide. They compound.

To put it simply, you are not just your race. Or just your gender. Or just your immigration status. You are *all* of those things at once. The way that society responds, judges, excludes, and/or elevates you happens at that intersection.[liii] Intersectionality helps us understand that identity isn't fragmented. My identity is not just a countertop full of ingredients and spices. I am all of the things that make Tony mixed together in a pot, like gumbo. When the world doesn't see the full you, it creates blind spots in how inclusion (or exclusion) is experienced.

In the context of imposter syndrome, that insight reveals something crucial. Self-doubt isn't always irrational. For people who live at the crossroads of multiple marginalized identities—say, a queer woman of color, or an immigrant with a disability—the voice that whispers, *you don't belong* isn't just in their head. It's being echoed by what they see and feel around them.[liv]

In many environments, we're underrepresented. Overlooked. Interrupted mid-sentence. We are expected to prove our worth, twice as hard half the time, and for less recognition. When someone is both a racial minority *and* a woman *and* an immigrant, the biases they face aren't just stacked. They are multiplied. The pressure to overperform becomes heavier. The cost of failure becomes steeper. The margin for error shrinks.

How many times have you felt that pressure yourself? You know, that "*I can't mess this up*" tension that sits in your chest. It is not because you're unsure of your skills. It's because you know one slip might confirm someone else's stereotype. That's not just fear. That's pattern recognition. You have seen it play out hundreds of times. You have already read this script and have seen this movie.

From this lens, imposter syndrome isn't just a psychological hurdle to clear with affirmations or regular confidence boosts. It's a survival strategy. A defense mechanism born from navigating systems that were never designed for people like you to lead, thrive, or to exist in.[lv]

And that brings us to Julissa.

Julissa's Story: The Voice Inside Her Accent

Jullisa is a proud Dominican woman who moved to Cleveland, Ohio, at sixteen after spending her childhood in the Dominican Republic. She's now a wife, a mother of three, a public servant, a graduate student, and a Harvard certificate candidate.

But even now, after all she's accomplished, she still doesn't always feel like she belongs in the spaces she's worked so hard to enter.

Her earliest ideas of what success looked like came through a tv screen. In the DR, while caring for her siblings in her mother's absence, she would watch American television. The women on those shows wore power suits. They gave orders. They were respected. They looked nothing like her. But they were everything she thought she wanted to be.

> *That's what success looks like, she thought. That's who I have to become.*

But success was not the world Julissa was born into.

When she was still a child, her mother left for the United States to receive cancer treatment, leaving Julissa and her siblings in the care of a family friend. Julissa, though the middle child, became the one who kept things together. She cooked, cleaned, woke her siblings up for school, mediated conflict, and tucked them in at night.

She was a child with an adult's responsibilities, and no space to fall apart.

By the time she was reunited with her mother and brought to Cleveland, six years had passed. Six years of learning not to cry. Not to need help. Not to expect things to be easy. She arrived in America already fluent in responsibility. But not English.

High school was lonely. Language isolated her. The other students didn't know how to make space for someone like her. And Julissa didn't know how to ask for it. So she stayed quiet—not because she had nothing to say, but because her voice didn't sound like theirs.

Even now, her accent remains. She speaks English fluently, with confidence and clarity, but the accent is still there. And it's not neutral. To Julissa, it feels like a warning bell.

They hear me before they see me. And once they hear me, they assume things. That I'm not as smart. That I'm not as prepared. That I don't really know what I'm doing.

She rehearses her thoughts before meetings. Proofreads emails three times. She overprepares because she knows there's less room for error. Because she believes, even now, that a single misstep could confirm what someone might already think: that she's not supposed to be there.

It's exhausting. Not just because of the labor, but because of the silence.

Don't mess up. Don't sound unsure. Don't let them think you're guessing—even when you are.

Still, she has climbed.

Julissa became the first in her family to graduate from college. She built a career in public service. She is pursuing her Master's Degree in Public Administration. She's enrolled in a certificate program at Harvard. She has raised three children. Maintained a marriage. Mentored others. And yet she still struggles to believe it's enough.

She dreams of becoming an immigration attorney. The calling is personal, rooted in her own family's journey, her understanding of the system, and her desire to advocate for those who feel voiceless. But even as she holds that dream, doubt shadows it.

I'm thirty-nine, can I really start over? Law school is hard. Expensive. Competitive. What if I'm not built for it? What if I fail?

She doesn't say these things out loud. For Julissa, strength has always meant pushing through without complaint. Even when the pushing becomes a quiet form of self-erasure.

She's also mapped out a nonprofit that would serve immigrant families. It's meaningful work. But she admits that it's her a backup plan. Just in case she never finds the courage to chase the thing she really wants.

What if I try and it doesn't work? What if I don't belong in those spaces, either?

But something in her is shifting. Slowly. She is beginning to speak to herself differently. To offer herself grace. To name the structures, not just the feelings.

"I'm learning to see my story as power," she says. "Even the parts that made me doubt myself."

Julissa is not just battling internal fears. She is navigating a society that rarely sees all of who she is. Her race. Her gender. Her accent. Her immigration story. Her motherhood. Her ambition. Her trauma. Her brilliance. These things don't cancel each other out. They collide.

And at that intersection is where her imposter syndrome lives.

Julissa's Story Is Intersectionality in Motion

Julissa doesn't suffer from imposter syndrome because she's insecure. She struggles because the systems she's succeeded in were not built for her to thrive. Her doubts are not delusions. They are shaped by a culture that consistently undervalues people like her.

She's not just a woman. Not just an immigrant. Not just a mother. Not just a student. She is all of those things at once. And every step forward has required her to navigate more than just the job in front of her. It has required her to carry and contend with the weight of her identity.

That is intersectionality in action.

And until we build systems that honor the full complexity of people like Julissa, imposter syndrome will continue to thrive. This is not because people lack confidence, but because they lack confirmation that they are welcome.

But Julissa is no longer waiting for confirmation. She's writing her own. And with every step she takes—into classrooms, boardrooms, courtrooms—she isn't just proving herself.

She's proving that power, in its truest form, is not about perfection, it is about presence.

Final Thoughts: Integrating Multiple Perspectives

The science behind imposter syndrome is complex, encompassing neurological responses, cognitive distortions, and systemic inequities. No single explanation is sufficient on its own. Understanding imposter syndrome requires an integrated approach that addresses both the internal and external factors that sustain it.

The chapters that follow will explore strategies that draw on each of these perspectives to help you dismantle self-doubt, embrace authenticity, and build unshakable confidence.

Chapter 6

Redefining Failure and Success

Introduction: How Imposter Syndrome Distorts Failure and Success

Imposter syndrome thrives on distorted perceptions of success and failure. These rigid, unrealistic standards leave no room for growth, learning, or the complexities of real life. For high achievers, success often means achieving perfection. Failure, even in its simplest form, equates to incompetence. This rigid thinking creates a relentless cycle of fear and self-doubt. This thinking makes it nearly impossible to embrace risks, pursue new opportunities, or acknowledge achievements as legitimate.

These distortions are not merely personal flaws. They are learned responses shaped by societal pressures, family expectations, and cultural narratives that equate self-worth with external achievements. From a young age, many high achievers internalize the idea that their value is conditional. It is directly tied to their last success and perpetually at risk of exposure if they somehow mess up and, heaven forbid, make a mistake. This creates a high-stakes reality where every mistake feels catastrophic and every success feels insufficient.

The real problem, however, may not be failure itself but the narrow, perfection-driven definitions of success that keep the stakes impossibly high. This chapter explores how imposter syndrome warps our understanding of success and failure. It explores how these definitions are both unsustainable and self-defeating. Further, it dives into how redefining these terms can free us from the cycle of self-doubt and perfectionism. Developing a more balanced view of success and a healthier attitude toward failure, allows us to create a more authentic and attainable foundation for true confidence.

The Dangers of All-or-Nothing Thinking

We talked about "all-or-nothing thinking" back in Chapter 2, but it's worth briefly revisiting here. It continues to shape how imposter syndrome distorts our understanding of success. This kind of thinking frames everything as either a win or a loss, a success or a failure. This way of thinking leaves no room for nuance. You're either exceptional or you're a fraud. There's no in-between.

Even when I know better, I still catch myself slipping into this mindset. If a project doesn't go exactly as planned, my first instinct isn't to reflect—it's to question whether I should've done it at all. This mental trap keeps us from acknowledging growth, because anything less than perfect doesn't count.

In the context of success and failure, all or nothing thinking turns progress into pressure. It strips away the possibility of learning through setbacks or celebrating partial wins. Combined with the moving goalpost effect, it becomes a recipe for burnout. You're chasing an ever-shifting definition of "enough." So, even if you hit it, it just does not feel like you found that success.

The Moving Goalpost Phenomenon: Why Success Never Feels Like Enough

The moving goalpost mindset is one of those traps that sneaks up on you. You hit a goal—maybe it's a degree, a promotion, or a big win—and instead of feeling proud, you instantly raise the bar. It's like, "Cool...what's next?" Before you've even had a chance to breathe, you're chasing the next milestone. And just like that, the thing you worked so hard for no longer feels like a success. It feels like the bare minimum.

This kind of thinking makes it nearly impossible to truly feel successful. You keep accomplishing more, but none of it sticks. There's always another bar to clear. And it's not just ambition. It becomes a cycle where every win is immediately dismissed as not enough. That pressure can show up in all kinds of ways. A professor publishes a major paper and instantly obsesses over getting the next grant. A newly promoted exec doesn't take a second to acknowledge the achievement, they're too busy trying to prove they deserve it.

Honestly, this isn't just self-inflicted. A lot of it is tied to how we're wired by culture, expectations, and this constant feeling that you've got to overperform just to be seen. The message is clear. *What you've done so far isn't enough to keep you in the room, let alone move you forward.*

Breaking out of this cycle takes work. It means slowing down enough to actually celebrate the wins, no matter how small. It means redefining success. It is not just how fast or far you go, but by how aligned it is with your values, your growth, and the impact you're making along the way.

This is intimately applicable to me. I am editing this book within two months of my official release of *Unlocking Potential*. Admittedly, simultaneously navigating the marketing journey for one book while writing and editing the second is overwhelming. Hopefully I will have resolved my "Moving Goalpost" issues prior to my next project.

As for today, I am still trying to navigate it like my friend Dr. Lisa Chang.

Dr. Lisa Chang's Story: The Chase for Validation That Never Ends

Lisa Chang had always believed that if she just achieved the next milestone, the doubt would finally disappear. If she got the degree, if she landed the right job, if she proved herself in every space she occupied—then, and only then, would she feel secure.

She had been chasing achievement for as long as she could remember. As a child of Chinese immigrants who had sacrificed everything for a better future, Lisa was taught that success wasn't optional. It was survival. Her father, a military veteran turned small business owner, reinforced the idea that education was the only way to ensure stability. She internalized this pressure early, convinced that she needed to prove that their sacrifices had been worth it.

When Lisa lost her mother at a young age, that pressure intensified. Her older brother, stepping into a caretaker role, urged her to focus on school as a way to create a different future. And she did. She excelled in academics. But the more she achieved, the less it felt like enough.

College should have been a time to celebrate her potential. Instead, college was where she first started moving the goalposts on herself. Enrolling at a large state university, she felt swallowed by the anonymity of giant lecture halls and the lack of structured guidance. Instead of acknowledging that she simply needed a better learning environment, she saw her struggle as proof that she wasn't good enough. When she transferred to a smaller liberal arts college and finally started thriving, she barely allowed herself to take credit for her intuition. *It's just because the classes are smaller,* she told herself. *It doesn't mean I actually belong.*

Lisa initially pursued a career in athletic training, but when she realized the financial instability of that path, she pivoted. With the encouragement of a mentor, she switched to community health and secured a graduate assistantship that paid for her master's degree. It was a clear victory, a sign that she was on the right path. But instead of feeling accomplished, she immediately started worrying about the next step.

If I really want to be taken seriously, I need more credentials, she thought.

That single thought set her on a path of endless striving.

Every time she reached a new level of success—whether it was landing a leadership role in nonprofit health, developing programs that impacted thousands, or securing millions in funding—she barely paused before raising the bar again. Her expertise was undeniable. Still, she constantly felt like she had to justify her place at the table.

*She believed he*r ultimate proof would come from earning a doctorate. *Once I have 'Dr.' in front of my name, then I'll feel legitimate*, she reassured herself. The logic seemed sound. A PhD was the highest credential in her field. Surely, that would silence the doubts.

It didn't.

Lisa poured years into earning her doctorate. She balanced research, work, and her personal life with the same relentless drive that had defined her career thus far. The moment she defended her dissertation and officially became Dr. Chang should have been one of triumph. Instead, the euphoria lasted mere hours before the doubt crept back in.

Well, it's just a title. It's not like I have as much experience as some of my colleagues. I probably need to get more articles published. Maybe I should look into another certification.

The goalposts had moved again.

Her breakthrough didn't come from another degree or title. It came from exhaustion. Lisa realized she was burning herself out chasing validation she would never let herself accept. The external milestones weren't the problem. It was her refusal to let them count.

So she made a shift. Instead of seeking success through endless credentials, she started measuring it by impact.

When she saw a young public health professional she had mentored secure her first major grant, she let herself feel pride—not just in that person's success but in her role in shaping it. When she built a program that changed the way health resources were distributed in underserved communities, she reminded herself that *this* was what mattered.

Lisa still fights the urge to move the goalposts. But now she recognizes it for what it is: a habit, not a necessity. She no longer believes that another degree, another title, or another project will finally make her feel like she belongs. Instead, she reminds herself that she already does.

By shifting her definition of success from constant achievement to lasting impact, Lisa has finally begun to break free from her moving goalpost phenomenon. And for the first time in her life, she's allowing herself to stand still long enough to appreciate how far she's come.

Creating a Personal Definition of Success

Society loves to measure success in titles, paychecks, plaques, and applause. Let's be honest, we like those things. Yet, those things can be loud, shiny, and often hollow. It creates this weird paradox that the more you achieve by those standards, the less connected you might feel to your own success. It starts to feel like you're chasing someone else's goals.

At some point, you've got to ask yourself, *what does success mean to me?* Not to your boss, your LinkedIn network, or your peers. What does it mean to you? Maybe success is having time to raise your kids without burning out. Maybe it's pouring into your community or mentoring the next wave of leaders. Maybe it is finally having the freedom to be creative without asking for permission or needing validation. It's different for everyone. The key is finding *your* definition.

Redefining success in your own terms doesn't mean lowering the bar. To the contrary, it means moving it to a place that actually reflects your values. It means shifting from a mindset that sees success as a final destination to a mindset that sees it as a journey. A journey full of growth, learning, and real impact.

When you do that—when your wins are aligned with what actually matters to you—confidence starts to feel less like a performance and more like a truth. And that kind of confidence lingers.

How High Achievers Can Learn from Setbacks

Failure is not the opposite of success. In fact, it is a crucial part of the growth process. Every successful person has experienced failures, setbacks, and outright defeats. What sets them apart is not an absence of failure but a willingness to learn from it. For high achievers struggling with imposter syndrome, reframing failure as feedback rather than a death sentence is essential.

The way you respond to failure often depends on how you understand growth. When you believe that your abilities can improve through effort and experience, mistakes start to feel like part of the journey; not a sign that you do not belong. This kind of thinking helps high achievers put failure in perspective. Imagine a startup founder whose product launch does not go as planned. Instead of seeing it as a personal failure, they treat it as useful information. They look at what went wrong, make adjustments, and try again. That mindset does not just protect your confidence, it builds resilience.

The key to learning from setbacks lies in analyzing what went wrong without attaching it to your self-worth. This means treating mistakes as opportunities for reflection, not as proof of inadequacy. By separating outcomes from identity, high achievers can build resilience, enhance their problem-solving skills, and transform failure from a source of self-doubt into a powerful tool for growth.

Turning Setbacks into Growth: Alex Harding's Journey

Alex Harding never imagined he'd end up practicing law. He was raised in Akron, Ohio, in a working-class family. Stability was their measure of success. Law school wasn't a foregone conclusion, it was an anomaly. He was the first in his family to graduate from college, and even then, he often wondered if he had simply outworked the system rather than belonged in it.

I'm smart...but maybe not that kind of smart.

That feeling was with him throughout undergrad. He drifted between majors before settling on political science. It was interesting enough, but uninspiring for a career after he graduated. He chose to go to law school. Not out of a deep sense of calling, but because it sounded like the next logical step. Something respectable. Something secure.

But once he got there, the insecurity intensified.

Legal writing was his Achilles' heel. Where others seemed to churn out polished drafts effortlessly, Alex labored over every sentence. He second-guessed punctuation, agonized over citations, and reread his work so many times it lost all meaning. Professors rarely offered praise, and when they did, he questioned whether they meant it.

> *Real lawyers don't struggle like this. If I can't master writing, what am I even doing here?*

His first legal job, a temporary clerkship, felt like confirmation of all his doubts. It should've been an easy stepping stone, but instead, it magnified the voice in his head that said he was a fluke. Every mistake felt enormous. Every red mark on a draft felt like proof that he didn't belong.

So when he transitioned into probate litigation, something shifted. The work was more structured, more form-based, more grounded in process than prose. And to his surprise, he liked it.

> *I'm not a wordsmith. But I can figure out the system. I can guide people through this.*

In probate, he found something that aligned with his strengths—his attention to detail, his empathy, his steady demeanor in moments of family crisis. But even then, the imposter syndrome lingered. He'd win cases, yet focus on the one sentence in a closing argument that hadn't landed. Clients praised him, but he'd brush it off as them being "just relieved it was over."

The next chapter of his career came at an elder law firm. Seemingly it was an upgrade. In reality, however, it felt quite hollow. The firm ran like a machine. Quantity over quality. Alex felt like a cog, churning out results that checked boxes but didn't deepen his understanding or feed his growth. The illusion of success was just that, an illusion.

> *Is this it? Am I going to spend my career doing work that looks good on paper but doesn't feel right in practice?*

He left. Quietly. Without a dramatic exit or a lined-up position. Starting his own practice wasn't a long-term dream, but survival. A leap into the unknown. Driven more by misalignment than ambition.

The early days were hard. He took on anything that came his way, including family law, landlord-tenant disputes, even a few messy personal injury cases. Every time he stepped outside his comfort zone, the old voice came back.

> *You're going to mess this up. And they'll finally see you for what you are.*

But each case taught him something. Not just about the law, but about himself. Slowly, he started to narrow his focus. He returned to probate work exclusively. Not because it was easy, but because it fit. It gave him room to be thoughtful. Strategic. Precise.

He created templates. Built systems. Focused on client education. He leaned into what worked for him (structure, preparation, and empathy) and let go of the need to be perfect in every other area.

Over time, the fear faded. Not entirely, but enough for him to send an invoice without feeling anxious about it. Enough to take a day off without guilt. Enough to mentor a younger attorney and actually believe he had something valuable to say.

Today, Alex Harding runs a thriving solo probate practice. He's no longer trying to prove he's smart enough to be a lawyer. He knows he is. He knows he has done the work. Not flawlessly, but consistently.

His story isn't about brilliance. It's about belief.

Maybe you don't need to write like a Supreme Court clerk. Maybe you just need to know who you are, what you bring, and trust that that's enough.

And for Alex, that's more than enough.

Final Thoughts: Failure as a Path to Growth

Imposter syndrome convinces us that failure is proof of inadequacy and that success must be flawless to count. But this mindset is both unsustainable and untrue. Failure is not only inevitable but necessary for growth. It teaches resilience, sharpens skills, and provides the kind of learning that no success alone can offer.

Reframing failure as part of the success journey rather than its opposite allows us to take risks, learn from mistakes, and keep moving forward without the paralyzing fear of being exposed as frauds. Success, in its truest form, is not about never falling down. It is about always getting back up, learning, adapting, and persisting.

By redefining success on your own terms, embracing failure as feedback, and breaking free from the moving goalpost and all-or-nothing thinking, it becomes possible to build a form of confidence that is both resilient and enduring.

Chapter 7

Confidence is Built, Not Inherited

Introduction: How Confidence is Built, Not Inherited

Confidence gets misunderstood all the time. We're taught to picture it as this loud, fearless, spotlight-stealing energy. As if you are always on. You are always the life of the party. If you don't naturally have that vibe, people tell you to "just fake it 'til you make it." Sure, that sounds good. That advice can do more harm than good. It makes it seem like confidence is something you're either born with or you're not. Like it's reserved for some chosen few who never question themselves. But that's not real life.

The truth is, confidence isn't magical. It's not a personality trait reserved for extroverts or overachievers. It's a skill. You can learn it. You can practice it. Over time, you can get better at it just like anything else.

A lot of high achievers get stuck in this weird in-between. If they admit doubt, they feel like frauds. But if they show confidence, they worry they'll come off as arrogant. If you've been through failure, rejection, or environments that made you second guess yourself, building confidence might feel even harder.

When your experiences have trained you to see risk as danger and mistakes as proof you're not good enough, it makes sense that you'd be on edge. Your brain learns that playing it safe feels better than putting yourself out there. That mindset can become your default if you're not careful.

But confidence isn't about knowing everything or never having fear. It's about trusting that you can handle whatever comes. It grows from showing up, making hard choices, and bouncing back when things don't go your way. It's about realizing you don't have to be perfect to be powerful. It's not the final destination. It's part of the process.

In this chapter, we'll look at how confidence is shaped by your experiences, how to rebuild it after hard seasons, and how to tell the difference between real self-belief and just trying to prove yourself to the world.

The Myth That Confidence Is "Innate"

Confidence is not about being fearless, never feeling self-doubt, or always having the right answer. Confidence is about trusting yourself to figure things out, even if you don't have all the answers yet. It is the belief that you are capable of handling challenges—not because you are guaranteed to succeed, but because you trust your ability to learn, adapt, and persist.

The myth that confidence is innate stems from a fundamental misunderstanding. Confidence is shaped through one's experiences. Positive experiences, such as mastering a skill, receiving encouragement, or achieving a difficult goal, serve as proof to your brain that you can handle what life throws your way. Negative experiences like failure, criticism, trauma, or environments that are harmful to your self-worth, can do the opposite. They train your brain to expect failure and interpret any setback as a sign that you are fundamentally incapable.

Building confidence lies in unlearning these false messages and replacing them with experiences that reinforce self-trust. This involves collecting small wins but also reframing how you interpret setbacks. Think of failures in a positive light. Look at it as if you are brave enough to try something new, even if you experience setbacks in the process. Confidence grows not from avoiding failure but from confronting it, learning from it, and choosing to move forward.

Redefining Success: Building Confidence on Your Own Terms

Traditional definitions of success—focused on external validation, perfectionism, and never-ending goalposts—fuel imposter syndrome. When success is defined by external markers such as titles, salaries, and accolades, it becomes fragile. A single failure or a critical comment can shatter your confidence because it feels like your entire worth is on the line.

When you define success based on your personal values, growth, and impact, your perspective of success changes. With that change in mindset, you see setbacks as growth as well, not as judgements against your competency and abilities. For instance, if you define success as continuous learning, then a failed project becomes a valuable lesson rather than proof of inadequacy. If success means making a meaningful impact, then it becomes less about the promotion you didn't get and more about how you contribute to your team's success each day.

The Role of Failure, Trauma, and Rejection in Confidence Development

Confidence is not built by avoiding failure but by learning to see failure differently. People often equate confidence with a perfect track record, but true confidence is about resilience. It is about your ability to recover, adapt, and move forward after setbacks. Each failure, rejection, or misstep is an opportunity to refine your skills, clarify your goals, and strengthen your emotional resilience.

However, for those who have experienced trauma, severe criticism, or unsupportive environments, the path to confidence can be more challenging. Trauma has a way of training your brain to hit the panic button even when there is no real danger. It wires you to see every risk as something to avoid, and every failure as a personal indictment. Over time, it becomes harder to separate real threats from old fears. So instead of stepping forward, you hesitate. Not because you are not capable, but because your brain has learned to treat discomfort like danger.

Building confidence in this context requires addressing both the psychological wounds of the past and creating new experiences of competence and safety. This might involve therapy to process past traumas, setting small and manageable challenges to build evidence of capability, and seeking environments that offer support rather than judgment. The goal is to rewire the brain's response to risk. This is not done by avoiding risk. You accomplish this by proving to yourself, incrementally, that failure is not fatal and that growth is possible even in the face of setbacks.

Confidence After Chaos: Layla's Story

Layla didn't learn confidence from comfort. She learned it from growing up in a world that demanded responsibility.

She was born and raised on the west side of New York City, a Puerto Rican girl in a neighborhood where resilience was the only real inheritance. Spanish was her first language, and it wasn't until the sixth grade that she began to speak English with any fluency. The shame she felt around her accent, the teasing from classmates, the silence she kept in class to avoid being laughed at, all laid the groundwork for a lifelong fear of being misunderstood, underestimated, or worse, dismissed.

At home, there was no refuge. Her mother was physically present, but emotionally unpredictable. Often angry. Often drinking. Her words came sharp and unfiltered, and rarely, if ever, affirming. Layla's father was a ghost, a name with no face, absent from her life but responsible for at least five other children she'd never met. Any ideas of safety or support had to be invented in her own mind, because they certainly weren't modeled around her.

Layla was the oldest, and from an early age, she became the caretaker. She cooked. Cleaned. Looked after her younger sister who, as an adult, now lives with a disability and struggles with substance use. That caretaking role never went away. Her sister now relies on social security and Layla's quiet, unwavering support. She's always been the one who holds it all together.

So when people see Layla now—successful, sharp, co-owner of a respected law firm, a public speaker with a growing YouTube following—they often assume she's always been this way. What they don't see are the layers of doubt she still carries. The way her voice still tightens before she speaks in front of an audience. The echo of the little girl inside her still asking, *Will they laugh if I get it wrong?*

When Trauma Becomes the Blueprint

Layla's relationship with confidence was shaped not by encouragement, but by adversity. She was cheated on, belittled, and abused in past relationships. She got pregnant young and feared, more than anything, that she might become her mother. She feared she would mimic the disconnected, overwhelmed, and emotionally volatile parent that she saw all of her life. Her sense of self-worth was constantly in question. And her fear of failure didn't stem from ego. It stemmed from the belief that failure would confirm what she'd long feared to be true. She did not belong in the spaces she was trying to enter.

Despite these fears, Layla worked for two decades as a paralegal. A steady and dependable role, which she excelled at. Yet the dream of becoming a lawyer remained quietly lodged inside her. Law school seemed impossible. Because of the cost, time, and risk, she convinced herself it was too late.

But eventually, something shifted. It wasn't a single moment of bravery. It was a gradual refusal to keep shrinking.

She applied. She enrolled. She studied while parenting, while working, while battling every insecurity that whispered she couldn't do it. She graduated as Cum Laude. She passed the bar. And has since soared.

The Ongoing Work of Believing You Belong

Layla didn't just become a lawyer, she stood out. In less than a decade, she moved from new associate to partner, then co-founded her own firm. She's built a platform for herself, becoming a sought-after speaker and content creator. She mentors other young women from marginalized communities. She leads with humility, empathy, and quiet fire.

But the trauma doesn't disappear just because the résumé shines.

Even now, before every keynote or interview, she still feels that familiar twinge of doubt. Her accent sometimes slips, and the old embarrassment bubbles up. She worries about being misunderstood. About not saying the "right thing." About not being enough.

But here's what's changed, she speaks anyway.

Healing Confidence Through Action

Confidence, for Layla, has been a daily decision. It has not been an inherited trait. It wasn't built through praise or perfect performance. It was forged through intentionality and persistence. Every time she raised her hand in law school, every client she represented, every courtroom she entered, she was building a case for her own belonging.

Layla continues to do the work of healing while building. She knows confidence is not about being fearless. It's about being willing to confront the fear. And she shows up, again and again, willing to grow through it.

She is not an imposter. She is the blueprint and is still building, brick by brick!

Confidence vs. Arrogance vs. Narcissism

Not all confidence is healthy. There is a significant difference between confidence, arrogance, and narcissism. Confidence is grounded in self-trust and self-awareness. Arrogance is rooted in a need to assert superiority. Narcissism is about controlling others to maintain an inflated self-image. Understanding these distinctions is crucial, especially in environments that often mistake arrogance for leadership potential.

Arrogance often masks deep insecurity. People who refuse to admit mistakes, dismiss feedback, or insist on being seen as superior are usually defending against self-doubt rather than expressing genuine confidence. This kind of false confidence is brittle. It tends to fall apart the moment it is challenged because it lacks the self-trust and resilience that define true confidence.

Layla has developed confidence. However, her humble spirit does not allow her to embrace arrogance or narcissism.

Genuine confidence, on the other hand, is about self-assurance without the need to prove anything to anyone. It's the ability to admit mistakes and learn from them. It is the ability to continue moving forward without the fear that one misstep will expose you as a fraud.

Building Confidence: Practical Strategies

Per Cuddy, confidence is a skill, which means it can be developed with practice. Practical strategies like visualization, intentional self-talk, and body language are grounded in neuroscience and psychology. In her book, *Presence*, Amy Cuddy (a social psychologist and Harvard researcher) discusses how confidence is not just an innate trait but a skill. This skill can be built through deliberate strategies like *power posing* (body language), *positive self-talk*, and *visualization*. She connects these practices to research in both psychology and neuroscience, showing that how we *act* can reshape how we *feel* internally over time.[lvi]

Visualization involves mentally rehearsing both the challenges and the desired outcomes. Intentional self-talk rewires the brain's default patterns from doubt to self-assurance. Body language influences how you feel and how others perceive you, creating a feedback loop that reinforces confidence.

The key is consistency. Confidence is not about grand gestures but about the small, repeated actions that build self-trust over time. It's about showing up even when you doubt yourself. Speaking up even when your voice shakes. Making decisions based on your values rather than your fears.

Final Thoughts: Confidence Is About Self-Trust, Not Perfection

Confidence isn't about being perfect or never feeling self-doubt. It's about trusting yourself to handle what comes your way. It is your ability to learn from failure, to adapt to uncertainty, and to keep moving forward. When you define success based on your values, growth, and impact, building confidence becomes a skill you can practice and strengthen over time.

In the next chapter, we will explore strategies for silencing the inner critic, managing overthinking, and transforming self-doubt into self-assurance. Confidence is not something you wait for. It is something you build. One small step at a time.

PART III

STRATEGIES FOR OVERCOMING IMPOSTER SYNDROME

Chapter 8

Owning Your Achievements

Introduction: Why Owning Your Achievements Matters

One of the most devastating effects of imposter syndrome is the inability to internalize success. High achievers often find themselves caught in a relentless cycle of dismissing their accomplishments. We attribute them to luck, timing, or the help of others rather than our own skills and hard work. This habit of downplaying success isn't just about modesty. It is a defense mechanism used to avoid the risk of being exposed as a fraud. However, the more we dismiss our achievements, the more we reinforce the belief that we don't deserve them. Over time, this erodes our self-confidence and deepens the sense of being a fraud. It is truly a vicious cycle.

Owning your achievements is not about arrogance or seeking validation. It is about reclaiming the narrative of your life from the grip of imposter syndrome. A narrative that insists no amount of success can prove your competence. Recognizing and celebrating your accomplishments builds a foundation of self-trust that makes it harder for self-doubt to take root. When we learn to see our achievements for what they truly are, evidence of effort, skill, and resilience, we begin to dismantle the false beliefs that keep us feeling like frauds.

This chapter explores why we minimize our success, the psychological and cultural factors that reinforce this tendency, and how to break free from these patterns. By learning to own our achievements without guilt or apology, we start to build more resilient and authentic confidence.

Why We Minimize Success and How to Stop

The habit of minimizing success often stems from a deep-seated fear of standing out. For many, acknowledging their achievements feels like inviting scrutiny or, worse, setting themselves up for failure. If you admit that you're good at what you do, what happens if you fail next time? This fear of being exposed as a fraud drives us to downplay our success and avoid drawing too much attention.

Another powerful factor is the fear of arrogance. Society frequently confuses confidence with conceit, particularly for women and marginalized groups. Women, for example, are often socialized to be agreeable and modest, to avoid being seen as "bossy" or self-serving. This conditioning leads to a reflexive habit of softening or deflecting praise with phrases like, "Oh, it was nothing," or "I just got lucky." The problem is that every time you dismiss your success, you reinforce the belief that you don't deserve it.

Breaking this habit requires practice. It means responding to praise with a simple "Thank you" and resisting the urge to downplay your contributions. Additionally, it means giving yourself permission to celebrate milestones, no matter how small. It reminds us that owning our success is not the same as boasting. It's about telling the truth about your life.

The Role of Humor and Self-Deprecation in Downplaying Success

Humor, particularly self-deprecating humor, is one of the most subtle but effective tools for deflecting praise. "Self-deprecating humor involves making oneself the target of a joke or playful criticism, often to appear humble, relatable, or to ease social tension."[lvii] By making a joke at your own expense, you can diffuse the discomfort of being complimented without outright rejecting the praise. It's a way of saying, "don't look too closely. I'm not really that great." For instance, when someone praises your leadership skills, you might respond with, "oh, I just play a boss on TV". Or, when complimented on a successful project, you might laugh it off as, "ha, I just fooled y'all again"!

Humor can serve as a useful coping mechanism in stressful situations. However, frequently using it to downplay success becomes a form of self-sabotage. By turning achievements into punchlines, you prevent yourself from internalizing them as real and earned. Over time, this can reinforce imposter syndrome, making it increasingly difficult to believe that you are competent.

The challenge is to find a balance. Humor can be a way to build rapport and show humility. It should not come at the expense of downplaying your capabilities. Again, simply accepting compliments without resorting to self-deprecating jokes can help you start to internalize success rather than dismiss it.

Reclaiming Your Accomplishments: Changing the Narrative

Reclaiming your achievements involves rewriting the stories you tell yourself about your success. This process starts by revisiting accomplishments you've dismissed or minimized. Make a list of ten achievements that you tend to downplay. These can range from career milestones, like securing a major client, to personal victories, like completing a challenging project or overcoming a significant setback. For each achievement, write down what made it possible. Identify what skills you used, the obstacles you overcame and the effort you invested.

For instance, if you led a successful project but have been telling yourself that it was only because you had a strong team, try reframing that narrative. Acknowledge that while having a capable team was an asset, your leadership, decision-making, and ability to coordinate efforts were what made that success possible. By breaking down the elements of your achievements, you transform them from lucky breaks into tangible evidence of your competence.

Another powerful technique for reclaiming accomplishments is to create a "Brag File". This is a collection of positive feedback, awards, emails of appreciation, or even notes to yourself about successes, both big and small. Whenever self-doubt creeps in, revisit this file. This is not about boasting, but about reminding yourself that your success is built on real skills and real work, not luck or deception. Over time, this practice trains your brain to see achievements as proof of capability rather than evidence of fraudulence.

Giving Others the Credit: A Way to Avoid the Spotlight

Another common tactic for downplaying success is deflecting credit onto others. It's true that most accomplishments are the result of collaborative efforts. Nonetheless, there is a difference between sharing credit and refusing to take any for yourself. For example, when praised for leading a successful project, someone struggling with imposter syndrome might immediately respond with, "Oh, it was all my team, they did the real work." While this instinct may seem humble, it can also be a way of avoiding the discomfort of acknowledging your own role in the success.

Jasmine Caldwell's career journey illustrates how this pattern can prevent individuals from fully stepping into their achievements.

Jasmine Caldwell's Story: A Reluctance to Own Success

Jasmine Caldwell had spent most of her career operating in the background, quietly contributing to impactful work while allowing others to take the credit. Raised in Charleston, South Carolina, she was the first college graduate in her immediate family. She earned a degree in political science, followed by a master's in public administration and a law degree. With each new accomplishment, she hoped she would finally feel like she belonged in professional spaces. Instead, she often found herself hesitant to fully own her expertise. This tendency followed her from government investigations to nonprofit work.

Jasmine's years as a federal government investigator were some of the most fulfilling of her career. The structured environment, clear responsibilities, and ability to work within established legal frameworks gave her confidence in her abilities. She was skilled at uncovering discrepancies, analyzing evidence, and drafting comprehensive reports. Yet, when commended for her work, she often dismissed the praise as "just following protocol" or "doing what anyone else would have done in my position."

Despite thriving in the role, the emotional toll of handling high-stakes cases led to burnout. She struggled to remain detached, feeling the weight of each investigation. Eventually, she left government work in search of a role where she could still make an impact without the constant emotional strain.

The transition reignited her imposter syndrome. Moving into advocacy and nonprofit policy work, Jasmine entered spaces dominated by PhDs in public health, many of whom had different credentials than hers. Though she had a legal and investigative background, she began questioning whether she was truly qualified to contribute at the same level. In meetings, rather than asserting her expertise, she would quietly pass notes to supervisors, suggest ideas privately, or downplay her role in shaping key initiatives.

Even when colleagues praised her for her insight, she instinctively shifted the credit elsewhere. If a policy recommendation she drafted gained traction, she would say, "oh, the leadership team really drove this forward." If a strategy she developed led to improved compliance, she would brush it off with "I was just lucky to be working with such a great team."

Her reluctance to acknowledge her own impact was not just about humility; it was about avoiding the pressure of being seen. She feared that if she fully owned her success, people would scrutinize her more closely, expecting her to deliver at an impossibly high standard every time. If she stayed in the background, she could contribute without the fear of being exposed as someone who didn't quite belong.

Reframing Success: Recognizing Your Role Without Diminishing Others

A healthier approach to success is acknowledging both the team's contributions and your own. For instance, instead of immediately shifting the spotlight onto others, you might say, "I had a great team, and I'm proud of what we accomplished together." This statement allows for shared recognition while reinforcing that your role in the success was real and valuable.

For Jasmine, breaking this habit has been a slow but intentional process. Now working in compliance and higher education, she is learning to step forward and own the work she has put in over the years. She no longer relies solely on private conversations to share her ideas. She speaks up in meetings. When she contributes to an impactful policy, she allows herself to say, "yes, I worked on that," instead of deflecting.

Her journey highlights a struggle many professionals face. The fear that claiming success will invite criticism or raise expectations too high is a real thing. The reality, however, is that refusing to acknowledge your achievements does not protect you from scrutiny. It only reinforces self-doubt.

Start with making small shifts in language. Respond to praise with a simple "thank you" instead of downplaying it. Or, document personal wins, no matter how small, in a journal. Leave notes on your fridge, affirming your progress. Small steps make it easier to internalize success as something earned, not borrowed.

Jasmine's story serves as a reminder. Owning your success does not mean taking credit from others. It means recognizing the truth of your contributions.

Final Thoughts: Embracing Your Success

Owning your achievements is about reclaiming the narrative of your life from the distortions of imposter syndrome. It is about recognizing that your success is not a fluke, not luck, but the result of your effort, skill, and perseverance. When you learn to embrace your achievements without guilt or apology, you build a foundation of confidence that is both authentic and resilient.

In the next chapter, we will explore strategies for silencing the inner critic and dismantling the self-doubt that fuels imposter syndrome. For now, give yourself permission to unapologetically own your success. Without qualification. Without apology. Without deflection.

Chapter 9

Silencing Your Inner Critic

Introduction: Understanding the Inner Critic

Everyone has an inner critic. It is the voice that amplifies flaws, questions your competence, and insists that you're not enough. For those grappling with imposter syndrome, this voice is especially damaging, turning every mistake into proof of incompetence and every success being luck. It thrives in high-pressure situations such as job interviews, leadership roles, or any moment that requires stepping outside your comfort zone. The inner critic's goal is to paralyze you with self-doubt, to keep you from taking risks that might lead to growth. It is the evil cousin to your inner voice that supports you and builds you up.

The truth is that your inner critic is not an unbiased observer. It exaggerates flaws, fixates on mistakes, and systematically ignores your strengths and accomplishments.[lviii] Understanding this voice—where it comes from, how it operates, and why it clings so desperately to its negative narrative—is the first step toward silencing it. In this chapter, we'll explore the origins of the inner critic, the cognitive distortions that fuel it, and practical strategies to transform it from a paralyzing enemy into a more balanced and constructive inner voice.

The Origins of the Inner Critic

That voice in your head? It usually isn't yours. The inner critic is a combination of people, moments, encounters, and experiences from your past. It's built from old comments, cultural messages, and painful memories. Those moments that hit harder than they probably should have. Most of the time, it starts when we're young. A parent who meant well but pushed too hard. A coach who only noticed you when you won. A teacher who pointed out every mistake but rarely praised your progress. Those moments stick. Little by little, they shape the voice you hear inside. It doesn't just push you to do better, but it beats you down when you don't. At some point, it stops being helpful and starts holding you hostage. It's not just holding you accountable. It is holding you back.

Those from historically marginalized backgrounds (Black and Brown people, women, LGBTQIA+ individuals, first-gen students and professionals) usually have a much louder inner critic. It's not just a voice rooted in personal memory. It's shaped by institutions, stereotypes, and repeated reminders. These factors, both overt and subtle, leave you to question your legitimacy. When you're always moving through spaces that don't fully see you or reflect who you are, the inner critic can start to feel less like self-doubt and more like self-protection. It becomes armor, or at least that is what you think. You brace for rejection before it even shows up. You question yourself before anyone else gets the chance to. It's like you try to beat them to the punch. *It won't hurt as much if I do it before someone else does.* But that kind of defense ends up doing more harm than good.

That's why for many high-achieving professionals from underrepresented communities, the inner critic is not just a voice of self-doubt. It becomes a survival mechanism. It critiques you before the world can and sharpens you before someone else tries to dull you.

When trauma and identity collide, the inner critic takes on a different role. It no longer just keeps tabs on how you're doing, it starts questioning whether you deserve to be here at all, by not only critiquing your performance, but also challenging your value. Dr. Elias Santiago knows this intimately.

Dr. Elias Santiago: A Voice Formed in Survival

Raised on the South Side of Chicago during the height of the crack epidemic, Elias came of age in an environment defined by instability, scarcity, and survival. His earliest memories were not of bedtime stories or birthday cakes, but of his mother struggling with addiction and the pain of his biological father being murdered. Love was there, but so was chaos. And so were the streets.

By middle school, Elias was hustling. First weed, then crack. Not because he wanted to destroy his life, but because he was trying to live it. He was trying to eat. Trying to be seen. Trying to matter. Trying to buy shoes and contribute to the bills. He wore confidence like a mask, but he barely made it out of high school with basic literacy. And soon, he found himself in front of a judge. He was now caught in a system that rarely grants mercy to young Black boys in sagging jeans and hand-me down trauma.

But that day, something rare happened.

The judge looked at him. She really looked at him. And instead of incarceration, she gave him probation. A second chance. An open door he didn't yet know how to walk through. All he knew was that he wouldn't waste it.

He made a promise that day—to the judge, to his grandmother, and to his mother—that he would finish school. He didn't know how long it would take, or if he was smart enough, but he gave his word. And for Elias, his word was holy.

He moved in with his grandmother. She fed him, clothed him, and gave him a quiet place to think. Meanwhile, his mother, who had once lived inside the storm of her own addiction, got clean. She earned her GED. They were healing on parallel tracks, pushing each other toward redemption with love and accountability.

Faith became the center of Elias's life. Deeply spiritual, he believed that his survival wasn't an accident. That God had not only preserved him, but expected something from him. That the promises he made were part of his covenant with both people and purpose. He enrolled at Harold Washington College. There, the professors saw more than a statistic, they saw a student. They helped him with bus passes, mentorship, and encouragement. They bought him a suit for interviews. One even gave him a credit card and said, "Don't let anything stop your journey."

And he didn't.

He earned his associate's degree. Then his bachelor's. Then his master's. Finally, he earned his Ph.D.

On paper, Dr. Elias Santiago is the embodiment of the American turnaround story. The streets-to-scholar pipeline. A success story you might read in a nonprofit annual report or see on a panel about resilience.

But paper doesn't tell you about the nights when he still doubts whether he belongs in the rooms he walks into.

The Inner Critic in Trauma's Shadow

Even now, with a doctorate and a respected academic position, Elias still hears the voice. Not all the time. But in certain moments, especially those moments he must be polished.

He remembers a night his insecurity surged. He was in a corporate suite at a White Sox game. A friend introduced him to a high-ranking executive, "this is Dr. Santiago," the friend proudly said.

But instead of standing tall at that moment, Elias shrunk on the inside. His thoughts scrambled. *What if they knew who I used to be? What if they don't believe this version of me is real? What if I lose it all?*

His shoulders tensed. His palms dampened. His breath tightened. The inner critic didn't care about his credentials. The inner critic reminded him of the courtroom. The basement. The trap house. The hunger. The shame.

That's what trauma-based imposter syndrome does. It doesn't ask for permission. It shows up in the very moments that should feel like triumph and turns them into tests. It asks questions laced with the past, *who do you think you are? What makes you think you belong here?*

But today, Elias knows how to answer it.

He breathes. He grounds himself in the facts, not the feelings. He reminds himself of the promises he made, and the man he became by keeping them. He doesn't fully silence the inner critic, but neither does he surrender to it. He recognizes it for what it is: a voice born from fear, not truth.

The same voice that once tried to keep him safe now tries to keep him small. But he's not small anymore. He's not a boy "begging for belonging." He's a man who "became who he said he would be."

And that is more powerful than any voice in his head.

Negative Self-Talk and Its Cognitive Distortions

Negative self-talk is the go-to language of the inner critic and it runs on cognitive distortions. We've already discussed the worst examples of cognitive distortions in chapter two with Izzy, including all-or-nothing thinking, catastrophizing, and discounting the positive. They'll have you blowing small mistakes out of proportion and brushing off your wins like they don't count. Little by little, they chip away at how you see your abilities and your worth. But once you learn to recognize these patterns, you can start challenging them. That's where real change begins.

Let's look at how that negative self-talk impacted Marcus Caldwell throughout his early career journey.

When Success Feels Conditional: Battling the Inner Critic

Raised in Cleveland, Ohio, Marcus was the eldest of seven siblings in a working-class household. His mother, who had him as a teenager, worked multiple jobs to provide for the family, often relying on Marcus to help manage the household. As a result, his childhood was marked more by responsibility than freedom. He spent his early years balancing school with the demands of co-parenting, often cooking meals, managing routines, and stepping in when his mother wasn't home.

Despite these challenges, Marcus excelled academically. He found refuge in school. His work ethic and intellect were rewarded there. He became a standout student and a natural leader, earning full scholarships to several universities. Eventually, he chose Bowling Green State University, influenced by a high school relationship. There, he quickly gained popularity and influence in student leadership circles.

But that early college success became a turning point. The discipline that carried him through high school gave way to overconfidence. He began skipping classes, deprioritizing academics, and underestimating how quickly small choices could snowball into larger consequences. What followed wasn't a dramatic failure, but a quiet unraveling. He landed himself a spot on the academic probation roster, and ultimately, was forced to leave school.

Returning home was devastating. With his mother now dealing with health issues and a recent divorce, Marcus felt an urgent need to contribute financially. Rather than returning to school, he went straight to work, taking on managerial roles in the corporate world and quickly rising through the ranks. On the surface, he was successful. He was well-paid, respected, and steadily building a career. But inside, he wrestled with a constant sense of inadequacy.

Entering corporate spaces without a completed degree made him hyper-aware of his perceived shortcomings. Surrounded by colleagues with formal credentials, Marcus began to question the legitimacy of his own accomplishments. He became increasingly cautious, believing that one misstep could expose him as a fraud.

He also struggled with minimizing his successes. Whether he was closing deals with major clients or being praised by executives, he often attributed it to luck or timing. He discounted the years of experience, the leadership he provided, and the work he put in.

The turning point came when Marcus began tracking his own success. A mentor had suggested that he reassess his successes. He started documenting client feedback, reviewing past projects, and noting key wins that reflected his value. Over time, this practice helped shift his thinking. He no longer relied solely on how he felt in a given moment. He began to rely on evidence.

Marcus's story is a powerful reminder that imposter syndrome is not always rooted in failure. Sometimes, it grows in the gap between what we've achieved and what we believe we're entitled to claim as success. Especially for those from working-class backgrounds, where success often feels precarious, that gap can be wide and persistent.

What helped Marcus wasn't just external validation. It was his intentional process of reframing his internal narrative. He didn't erase the past. He rewrote how it lived in him.

And in doing so, he gave himself permission to see his success as real, earned, and worthy of pride.

Transforming the Inner Critic into an Inner Coach

Silencing your inner critic doesn't mean eliminating self-reflection. Constructive self-reflection lets you recognize where you can grow without tearing yourself down or questioning your value. This shift involves transforming the critic into a coach. Allow it to become a voice that points out weaknesses as opportunities for growth rather than as evidence of incompetence.

To make this shift, practice responding to your inner critic with questions rather than condemnation. When it insists that you're not qualified, ask, "what skills can I improve to feel more confident in this role?"This reframes criticism as a call to action rather than a verdict on your worth.

Visualization can also help. Picture your inner coach as a mentor who believes in your potential. It becomes someone who balances feedback with encouragement. By consciously practicing this mindset, you train your brain to interpret setbacks as part of the learning process rather than as confirmations of inadequacy.

Reclaiming the Narrative: Techniques for Challenging Negative Thoughts

Transforming your inner critic takes more than just telling yourself to think positively. It starts with building awareness and following it up with intentional action. The first step is to notice when negative self-talk creeps in, and then resist the urge to believe it without question. For example, if a thought like *I'll never get this promotion* pops up, pause and ask yourself, "what's really going on?" Are you falling into all-or-nothing thinking, catastrophizing, or assuming you know what others are thinking?[lix] Recognizing the distortion is powerful because it allows you to step back and see how your thoughts might be exaggerating the truth.[lx]

After you've identified the distortion, the next step is to reframe it. Swap out something like "I'm terrible at this" with "I'm still learning, and I'm making progress." Reframing doesn't mean pretending everything is perfect. It means choosing a more honest and balanced way of thinking, one that acknowledges your effort and growth without tearing you down.[lxi]

Another helpful practice is journaling. Putting your thoughts on paper gives you the chance to examine them more closely. It turns abstract fears into something concrete that you can look at, question, and challenge.[lxii] Try using prompts like *"what proof do I have for this thought?"* or *"what would I say to a friend if they felt this way?"* These simple questions can shift your perspective and help quiet the inner critic. Journaling gives shape to the noise in your head and gives you the space to take back control of the story you're telling yourself.

Final Thoughts: Confidence as a Choice, Not a Feeling

Silencing your inner critic is not about eradicating self-doubt but about refusing to let it dictate your actions. Confidence isn't the absence of doubt. It's the decision to act despite it. When you transform your inner critic into an inner coach, you build a foundation of self-trust that can withstand setbacks and failures.

In the next chapter, we'll explore how to take up space confidently, advocate for yourself, and show up in both personal and professional environments with authenticity and assurance. For now, focus on recognizing your inner critic for what it is. A voice of fear, not a voice of truth.

Chapter 10

Mentorship, Representation & Community

Introduction: Why Mentorship Matters in Overcoming Imposter Syndrome

Imposter syndrome tends to grow when you're isolated. When you believe that your doubts and struggles are yours alone, it becomes easier to think you are the only one who does not belong. You start to feel like everyone else is confident, capable, and moving forward while you are pretending to keep up. *Maybe I am the only one who feels this out of place.* Mentorship can disrupt that narrative. The right mentor helps you see that even people who seem successful have wrestled with the same doubts. What you are feeling is not failure. It is a part of the process.

For many, mentorship is the first space where your inner struggles are seen but not judged. It is where someone with more experience can say, "you are not the only one who has felt this way. You are not broken. You belong." That message can be a turning point. It can mean the difference between stepping away or stepping up, between staying small or taking the risk to grow. Sometimes, that one conversation is what pulls you back from the edge.

Mentorship is not a one-sided relationship where advice only flows in one direction. At its best, it is a real connection that pushes you to see more in yourself. A good mentor does not just give you career advice. They help you quiet the noise of self-doubt, challenge the lies you tell yourself, and remind you of your value when you are tempted to forget it. *You are capable. You just needed someone to hold up a mirror long enough for you to see it.*

One person who experienced this firsthand is Malcolm Carter, a man whose outward confidence masked years of deep-seated imposter syndrome.

Mentorship as a Mirror: Malcolm Carter's Story

Malcolm Carter is the type of man who walks into a room and owns it. His handshake is firm, his voice steady, his presence magnetic. To anyone watching, he radiates confidence, the kind that makes people lean in and listen. But beneath the polished exterior, Malcolm spent years feeling like he was faking it, terrified that someone would expose him.

Raised by a single mother in Cleveland, Ohio, Malcolm learned early that confidence wasn't just a trait, it was a tool for survival. His mother, who worked multiple jobs to provide for her children, instilled in him the belief that the world would try to undermine him. "Never let them see you sweat," she told him. That mantra became his armor.

Through high school and college, Malcolm used charisma and humor to navigate spaces that felt foreign to him. At the University of Akron, he joined a Black Greek-letter organization, where he learned the art of networking, commanding a room, and speaking with authority, even when he didn't feel it inside.

But as he stepped into corporate spaces, imposter syndrome took hold. In his first professional job, on his very first day, his white supervisor casually offered him donated suits from a clothing closet. She assumed he couldn't afford professional attire. Malcolm smiled and declined politely, but inside, the comment stung. No matter how polished he looked, some people would always see him as less than.

The defining moment came when he was invited to speak at a high-level business council meeting filled with executives and CEOs. Though he was the expert in the room, his confidence wavered as he stepped up to the podium. *What if they realize I don't belong? What if I say something wrong?*

Sensing his hesitation, a mentor—a senior colleague—leaned over and said, "they don't know what you don't know. You define the situation, not the other way around."

That moment shifted something in Malcolm. Confidence wasn't about knowing everything. It was about owning what he knew. He delivered the rest of the presentation with authority, realizing that expertise isn't about perfection, but about trusting yourself to adapt.

Over the years, Malcolm's mentors helped him dismantle his imposter syndrome, reminding him that his presence in these spaces wasn't accidental, it was earned. Now, as a mentor himself, he teaches young Black professionals what he once struggled to believe. Belonging isn't something you wait for, it's something you claim.

The Different Types of Mentors and How They Help

There is no single type of mentor who can meet every need. In reality, different types of mentors serve distinct roles in your development, each offering unique forms of support that can help dismantle imposter syndrome. Strive to cultivate a diverse mentorship circle that includes peers, industry veterans, encouragers, and "unofficial" mentors that you observe from afar. This creates a diverse and powerful network of support, perspective, and guidance.

But how do you find these mentors, especially when you believe that you're not worthy of their time or attention? The answer lies in shifting your mindset about mentorship from something that you earn to something that everyone deserves in the pursuit of growth. Additionally, it involves embracing vulnerability by being transparent about your struggles and areas where you seek guidance.

The Peer Mentor: The Companion on the Journey

Peer mentors often get overlooked because they do not look like the mentors we usually imagine. They are not ten steps ahead with decades of experience. They are right there with you or maybe just a little further down the path. But that is exactly what makes them valuable. They understand what you are facing, not from memory, but because they are walking through it too.

What makes peer mentorship powerful is the way it makes the struggle feel normal. It is more relatable. Someone at your level admitting that they are figuring it out as they go, or that they also question if they belong, takes some of the sting out of self-doubt. You stop feeling like you are the only one trying to hold it all together. That kind of connection creates space to be honest about your fears without worrying that you will be seen as weak or unprepared. And sometimes, just knowing you are not the only one navigating the mess is enough to keep going.

Being honest with a peer mentor about your insecurities can feel uncomfortable at first, but more often than not, it brings relief. You realize you are not the only one carrying those doubts. You do not have to start with anything heavy. Just keep it real. Be honest, say something like, "lately I have been questioning whether I truly belong in this role. Do you ever feel that way?" That kind of openness invites connection. It allows the other person to let their guard down too, and what starts as a vulnerable moment often turns into one of the most honest and supportive parts of the relationship.

The Industry Guide: The Strategic Navigator

An industry guide is the kind of mentor who helps you see the bigger picture. They are not just focused on where you are right now but are thinking about where you are going. They understand the unwritten rules, the long game, and the moves that shape a lasting career. While a peer mentor might connect with your current experiences, an industry guide brings clarity about what lies ahead. They help you navigate power structures, identify meaningful opportunities, and make decisions that align with your purpose and growth.

Having this kind of support can be a game changer. When someone with real experience and credibility sees something in you, it challenges the belief that you do not belong. Their belief in your value becomes a counterweight to your doubt. It reminds you that what you bring to the table matters and that you are not invisible to the people who understand the work best.

Opening up to an industry guide does not usually happen right away. It takes time for that kind of relationship to build. Being vulnerable with someone who has so much experience can feel intimidating. In the beginning, it is natural to want to prove yourself and keep up the appearance that you have everything together. But as trust grows, so does the opportunity for real connection. Eventually, there may come a moment when you feel ready to say what you have been carrying quietly. You might share that you value their insight but sometimes question whether you truly measure up.

That kind of honesty can shift everything. It helps your mentor understand how to support you more deeply, and shows that you trust them enough to be real. These moments are often where the mentorship becomes more than just career advice. They are where growth begins, both professionally and personally.

Scott: What did he see in me?

Scott Whitman didn't expect to become a bureau manager. For a long time, he didn't even expect to become steady. His early years in Cleveland were messy, Full of movement, full of anger, full of moments that could have derailed him completely. He didn't have a blueprint. No college degree. No long-term plan. Just a knack for figuring things out on the fly and a quiet fear of being found out.

He knew he was smart. He knew he could outwork just about anyone. But even as he moved up through demolition work, then construction inspection, then certification, something always tugged at him, *you didn't come in the right way. They'll realize it eventually.*

The voice was always there, especially in boardrooms and planning meetings. Especially when titles started mattering more than know-how. It was imposter syndrome, though Scott wouldn't have used that language back then. For him, it just felt like walking on eggshells in steel-toe boots.

Then he met Tom.

Tom was a 20-year veteran in city government. Respected. Straight shooter. Not flashy, but sharp. The kind of guy who knew how to read a blueprint and a politician with the same precision. When Tom joined Scott's division as a senior advisor, most people thought he'd be too far up the ladder to care about the new guy climbing behind him.

But Tom saw something.

At first, their conversations were mostly technical. Regulations. Permits. Field reports. But over time, Tom started pulling Scott into bigger rooms such as economic development calls, infrastructure meetings, budget forecasts, etc. He didn't just want Scott to know his own job. He wanted him to see the full "chess board."

"You've got the instincts," Tom told him one afternoon. "But you've got to stop acting like you snuck in through the side door. You belong here. You know how I know? Because if you didn't, I wouldn't waste my time."

Scott laughed nervously, brushing it off. But something about the way Tom said it stuck. It was the first time someone at that level had looked him in the eye and not just seen potential, but respected him.

If he sees it, maybe it's real. Maybe I'm not faking it.

Tom became more than a supervisor. He became an Industry Guide for Scott. A mentor that offered both insight and vision. He didn't coddle. He didn't flatter him. He challenged Scott to think beyond the next certification or promotion.

"You need to stop solving today's problems like it was five years ago," Tom once said. "Start playing a longer game. Think three years ahead, not three weeks."

At first, Scott was hesitant to be vulnerable. The years had trained him to play things close to the chest. But one day, after botching a presentation he'd spent hours preparing, he found himself blurting it out:

"I don't know if I can keep up with this level. I still feel like the kid who didn't finish school. Like I'm not allowed to mess up."

Tom didn't blink.

"You know what I used to feel," he said? "Like I'd be found out for not knowing enough. But the truth is, nobody knows everything. What sets you apart is that you don't stop asking. You don't coast. That's not weakness, that's how leadership's built."

That conversation shifted something. Scott started opening up more about what he didn't know. He became more transparent about how he wanted to grow in his career. About the fear that failure wouldn't just sting, it would confirm every doubt he had about himself.

Tom never made him feel foolish for it. Instead, he started helping Scott see his own career as a narrative. It was not just a series of jobs. It is a story with structure, setbacks, and strategy.

He helped him get comfortable not just with competence, but with vision.

"He made me stop thinking like a technician," Scott says now. "And start thinking like a leader."

And the more Scott owned that role, the quieter the inner critic became.

Imposter syndrome didn't vanish. But it lost its power. Because now, every time it whispered, *you don't belong here,* Scott had a voice louder than doubt reminding him, *you've earned every seat you sit in. Act like it.*

The Encourager: The Confidence Builder

While industry guides offer strategy, encouragers offer strength. Their focus is not on long-term strategy but on mindset and emotional resilience. They are the mentors who remind you of your strengths when your inner critic is loudest. They help you find balance against the tendency to fixate on flaws and dismiss achievements.

Encouragers are particularly receptive to honesty about insecurities. When you're candid about your struggles, they can provide more targeted support. Saying something like, "I've been really doubting my abilities lately and could use some perspective," opens the door for them to counteract the distorted self-talk that fuels imposter syndrome.

Starting Over Twice—The Path of a First-Generation Attorney

Attorney Lisa Moore grew up in the Midwest, between Indiana and Michigan in a home marked by instability. Her early years were punctuated by constant transitions. Her mother was neither nurturing, nor always there. She bounced between multiple schools, encountered strained family dynamics, and emotional whiplash from a biological father who was in and out of her life. Couple that with a domestic violence arrest as a teen for punching her mother's husband in the face.

There was only one stable person in her life, Raymond. He took Lisa in after she had to leave her mother's house when she struck her mother's husband. Raymond, the man she calls her "adoptive dad" never legally adopted her but he showed up. He showed up with groceries when she was broke. With encouragement when she doubted herself. With a steadiness she couldn't always find in her biological family.

"He didn't owe me anything," she would later reflect. "But he gave me everything he could."

None of the adults around Lisa had college degrees. Her biological father dropped out in ninth grade. Her adoptive dad and her mother both finished high school, but that was it. Lisa was the first in her family to go to college. The first to pursue a professional career. The first to imagine herself as something more than what she'd seen growing up.

And yet, despite all her credentials (honors student, varsity athlete, 4-H president, debate team captain) Lisa still walked through her world convinced that the next door might not open.

What if I'm not supposed to be here? What if I was just lucky?

The Law School Collapse

After graduating from college with honors, Lisa chose Charlotte School of Law because it offered her a scholarship. She was a first-generation student and no one had taught her how to pick a law school. So when someone finally offered her a way in, she took it.

The school soon became a disaster.

Behind the scenes, Charlotte School of Law was operating under federal scrutiny. It used a harsh academic curve to force students out of their scholarships. By Lisa's third year, just months before graduation, the school lost its federal funding.

I could finish here and graduate from a school that might not exist a year from now, she thought, *or I could walk away and start over.*

She walked away.

She packed up her apartment, moved to Ohio, and restarted law school. She lost more than a year's worth of credits in the process. Although it was the right decision, that decision haunted her.

It felt like a failure. Like I'd already proven I wasn't smart enough to pick the right path.

When she enrolled in her new program, she kept a low profile. She didn't want to explain her transfer. She didn't want people to ask questions. She felt like a warning sign in every classroom.

Learning to Belong

But Lisa made a quiet decision. If she had to start over, she was going to do it right.

She joined the moot court team. She became vice president of the Women's Law Student Association. She worked internships. She studied with her classmates. She figured out what kind of lawyer she wanted to be.

Public defense surprised her. At first, she imagined herself in family law. Maybe she would work with children like the girl she used to be. The lost, overlooked, and hurting. But once she stepped into the world of indigent defense, something clicked.

This is where I can fight for people who never had someone fighting for them.

After finally graduating with honors, she opened her own law practice. Her first big case was a rape charge, after having only been practicing for one month.

I have no business doing this, she told herself. *This isn't imposter syndrome. This is just reality.*

She picked up the phone, searching for someone who could take the case off her hands. That's when she met Derek.

The Power of a Peer Mentor

Derek had over a decade of experience and a reputation for excellence. But more importantly, he listened. He taught. He encouraged her.

Lisa no longer wanted to hand off the case, she wanted to work it with him. That case became the foundation of an unspoken mentorship.

Whenever Lisa second-guessed herself, she called Derek.

She remembers one moment vividly. It was an OVI (Operating a Vehicle while Impaired) case. The plea offer was standard. Everyone told her to take it. But Lisa had filed a motion to suppress and believed she had grounds to fight.

Why is everyone telling me to settle? she wondered. *Do they know something I don't?* Derek reminded her, "you know the case better than anyone. Trust yourself."

That advice stayed with her.

He became her quiet compass, not just for the law, but for her belief in herself. In those moments when the internal critic screamed *you're going to screw this up,* Derek's mentorship served as the rebuttal.

Derek was more than a guide. He was her Encourager. When Lisa's confidence wavered, he didn't just offer legal analysis. He affirmed her instincts, reminded her of her strengths, and countered the self-doubt she hadn't yet learned to silence. His mentorship didn't just sharpen her legal skills, it strengthened her emotional resilience.

More Than One Encourager

Lisa's growth wasn't built on the shoulders of one mentor. In addition to Derek, she connected with a federal public defender through Gideon's Promise—a national program for public defenders. That mentor, based in Georgia, remains a consistent source of wisdom.

They exchange texts often. Lisa always sends a picture of her son first, that's their inside running joke. "Here's the Mason text," she'll say, before asking for help. He is so cute that she cannot refuse Lisa's requests. Their relationship is one of mutual respect and authenticity. It's that authenticity that has helped Lisa speak her doubt aloud. She doesn't have to pretend with her mentors. She doesn't hide the fear. She can be vulnerable and transparent.

"I've been really doubting my abilities lately. I feel like I'm not measuring up", she once confessed during a call.

They didn't rush to fix it. They reminded her of her strength.

Encouragers don't make the fear disappear. They just make sure it doesn't win.

Final Reflections

Lisa is still a public defender. She doesn't make a corporate salary. She doesn't wear designer suits. She doesn't have THE corner office.

But she has a purpose. She has an impact. Slowly, she's learning to believe that she belongs.

"I used to think being a lawyer meant being perfect. Now I know it means being present. It means showing up, even when you're scared. It means using your voice for someone who doesn't have one."

She's not done fighting her imposter syndrome. But she's no longer doing it alone.

The Unofficial Mentor: Learning by Observation

Not all mentorships are formal. Unofficial mentors are those whose careers you admire from afar. You study their work. You trace their path, even if you never exchange a single conversation. You learn from them by observing how they navigate challenges, advocate for themselves, and balance confidence with humility.

An unofficial mentor serves as living proof that success does not require perfection. By following their journeys, including their missteps, pivots, and recoveries, you gain a more nuanced understanding of what success actually looks like. This perspective challenges the myth that everyone else has it all figured out, making it easier to embrace your own imperfect path.

My Story, Continued: Reflection on Dr. Jimmy Gray

I found an unofficial mentor in one of my fraternity brothers, Dr. Jimmie Gray. I met Jimmy at the gym over a decade ago. We learned that we were frat brothers quickly and would work out together from time to time. The mentorship would come years later. Honestly I do not recall how it did, I just recalled asking Jimmy if we could connect for some wings and drinks. We kept those sporadic meetings up for years, learning more about his 9-5 with the Federal Reserve in Cleveland, Ohio. More interesting to me was his 5-9 role as a business consultant with his company, Gray Management. Further, Jimmie is a published author, having written *Leadership in Action* as well as the companion workbook.

Dr. Gray has been an invaluable example to me of how to still be the "Owt Bruhs." But, most importantly, he has been an example of someone that matured in his career through continued education, discipline to write a book and the conviction to stay in good physical health. Last, but far from least, he has been an example through his determination to work throughout the day and commit to a thriving practice at night. Having him as a mentor has

145

been invaluable in helping me realize that I can do these audacious things also. Thanks Jimmie!

Representation and Its Role in Building Confidence

Representation is not just about being seen. It is about being affirmed. When you see someone who shares your background, your identity, or your lived experience in a position of influence, it sends a message that success is not limited to one kind of person. It pushes back against the quiet voice that tells you that you do not belong. It gives your inner critic something to confront. It provides concrete evidence that people like you can and do succeed.

For people from marginalized communities, whether that means race, gender, sexuality, or ability, representation holds even more weight. Without it, imposter syndrome can settle in and stay. When you rarely see people who look like you or live like you in leadership roles or respected spaces, it becomes easy to believe the lie that you are the exception instead of the expectation.

Think back to Malcolm from earlier in this chapter. Being the only Black man in the room made his imposter syndrome feel heavier. But when he connected with mentors who had faced the same challenges, something shifted. It was not just about seeing others, but about seeing himself reflected in their journey. That is what representation does. It does more than open doors. It helps you believe you belong on the other side of them.

Building a Community That Reinforces Belonging

Imposter syndrome is most difficult to manage when you feel like you are dealing with it alone. That is why mentorship and representation need to be backed by a real community. Your village! Having a group of people who see you, understand your journey, and affirm your growth creates a sense of belonging that can quiet the internal doubts. Whether it is through a professional network, an affinity group, or a small circle of peers. Those spaces help remind you that your success is not a mistake.

Look for communities that reflect your values and goals. Join groups that align with your identity. Show up to events that interest you. Take the time to connect with people who feel like a good fit. Building those relationships is not always quick, but it is worth it. Over time, those connections offer something that isolation never can. They provide support, accountability, and real validation.

Being around people who believe in you and understand your path can shift your perspective. It helps you see that you are not the only one figuring things out, and you do not have to prove your worth alone. Sometimes just knowing you are part of something bigger is enough to help you keep moving forward.

Final Thoughts: Mentorship, Representation, and Community as Acts of Resistance

In a world that can make you second-guess whether you belong, building relationships with mentors, role models, and a supportive community is more than just guidance. It becomes a way to reclaim your space and remind yourself that you have every right to be there.

The next chapter will dive into what it means to take up space with confidence, especially in environments that may not feel built for you. But for now, focus on the relationships that help you grow. Surround yourself with people who see your value, speak life into your goals, and remind you that your place at the table is not just earned, it is necessary.

Chapter 11
Thriving in High-Stakes Careers

Introduction: The Unique Pressures of High-Stakes Careers

areers that come with high levels of pressure demand precision, quick thinking, and strong decision making. For many professionals in fields like law, medicine, finance, technology, and politics, the expectation to perform at a high level without error is constant. These are not environments where small mistakes go unnoticed. The consequences can be serious, ranging from financial fallout and public criticism to legal risk or even the difference between life and death. For high achievers who already lean toward self-doubt or perfectionism, this pressure can push imposter syndrome to overwhelming levels.[lxiii]

What makes this dynamic even more complex is the irony that the very traits that drive success, discipline, attention to detail, and high standards can also become internal traps. Constant exposure, visibility, and comparison to others in competitive spaces create fertile ground for self-doubt to grow. "The more accomplished you are, the more likely you are to feel like a fraud."[lxiv] Navigating these pressures without letting every misstep define your worth is essential if you want to maintain confidence and protect your well-being.

This chapter looks closely at why imposter syndrome can feel especially intense in demanding careers. It offers strategies for managing that pressure, developing confidence that is grounded rather than performative, and setting limits that protect your energy and focus. It also explores the important role that therapists, coaches, and trusted advisors can play in helping professionals thrive without burning out.

Healing Others, Questioning Herself: The Silent Strain of Imposter Syndrome

In high-stakes careers, where the margin for error is slim and the consequences of mistakes are severe, imposter syndrome thrives. For Maya Ellis, a young Black nurse who quickly rose to a leadership role at a Veteran's hospital, the pressure was relentless. As the youngest nurse manager in her unit, Maya was responsible for decisions that directly impacted patient care and staff safety, particularly during the COVID-19 pandemic. The stakes were not just professional but personal. Every decision felt like a test of her worth.

One of the most pervasive myths in high-stakes careers is the idea that leaders must project unshakable authority. They strive to never show uncertainty. They never hesitate. They never admit what they don't know. For Maya, this myth was both a burden and a trap. As a young Black woman in a leadership role, she felt the pressure to appear twice as competent as her white counterparts just to be seen as credible.

The fear of failing was compounded by financial pressures that had haunted her since nursing school. Growing up, Maya's family had sacrificed so much to get her to this point. The thought of wasting her's and their efforts was paralyzing. Nights before exams, she would lie awake, the ceiling blurred by tears. She would replay every sacrifice her parents had made. She could still see her mother's hands, calloused and dry from years of handling chemicals in the lab, packing lunches to save money. The guilt was suffocating.

Maya's father, a retired Marine, was her anchor. Whenever the weight of expectations became too much, she would call him, her voice small and cracking. His advice was simple, "focus on what you can control." In one call, when she admitted to feeling like a fraud, he paused and said, "if you were a fraud, you wouldn't be worried about doing it right. Frauds don't care if they mess up." The words were a lifeline, pulling her back from the spiral of self-doubt.

But even with her father's support, Maya could not escape the loneliness of being one of the few Black women in leadership at her hospital. In a room full of white doctors and nurses, her voice always seemed too loud, her confidence too presumptuous. She felt the unspoken question, "what is she doing here?" hang heavy in every staff meeting. During one particularly tense meeting about COVID protocols, Maya felt her hands tremble as she spoke, watching older, white colleagues exchange glances.

When one doctor sighed audibly, her throat tightened, and she finished her presentation with her nails digging into her palms, leaving crescent-shaped imprints.

The institutional racism embedded in the hospital amplified her self-doubt. Her achievements were often dismissed as luck or lowered standards, making it almost impossible to internalize any success. When her supervisor offhandedly remarked, "we need more diversity, so this promotion is good optics," Maya smiled tightly, but inside, the words burned. If her successes were just about optics, then every late night, sacrificed weekend, and decision made under pressure meant nothing.

Staff meetings became exercises in code-switching. Maya found herself adjusting her tone, softening her voice, and choosing her words with surgical precision to avoid being labeled as angry or emotional. She would rehearse phrases in her head. Consistently she would rephrase directives as suggestions and mask any assertiveness with a smile. She recalls another deflating experience where her suggestions were dismissed until a white colleague repeated them verbatim. Maya locked herself in the bathroom and stared at her reflection, biting back tears of frustration.

Perpetual Comparison to High-Performing Peers

In high-stakes fields, the standard of success is often set by the top 1%. They are the outliers whose achievements are not just impressive, but unattainable for most. For Maya, this culture of perpetual comparison was suffocating. Even as she implemented successful initiatives

, it never felt like enough. Success was always moving goalposts. If it wasn't perfect, it didn't count.

Scrolling through LinkedIn became a nightly ritual of self-loathing. Former classmates posted about promotions, publications, and accolades with photos of white coats and wide smiles. Their successes seemed effortless, making Maya's own struggles feel like proof of failure. She would close the app with a heavy chest, her mind a litany of accusations. *They're doing all of that without burnout. Maybe I'm just not cut out for this.*

The pressure wasn't just external. Maya often found herself comparing her achievements to her mother's career in microbiology. Whenever her mother spoke about discovering a new bacterial strain, Maya's pride was eclipsed by a nagging voice that whispered, *She did that with three kids and no help. What's your excuse?*

The Fear of Costly Mistakes

The fear of making mistakes is not just a byproduct of high standards. It is a reflection of the real risks involved. For Maya, the fear of mistakes was a constant shadow. As a nurse manager during the pandemic, a single oversight could lead to exposure, illness, or even death among her team or patients. The pressure created a risk-averse mindset where even minor errors felt catastrophic.

One particular incident haunted her. During the height of the pandemic, a delay in ordering Personal Protective Equipment (PPE) due to hesitation over the correct protocol, left her team exposed for an extra day. This, unfortunately, resulted in an investigation. No one fell ill, but Maya spent weeks replaying the decision in her mind, convinced it was proof of her inadequacy. She could barely look her team in the eye, convinced they saw her as incompetent. The guilt was relentless, bleeding into her sleep. Nightmares of empty supply closets and gasping patients left her waking up in cold sweats.

Maya's aunt, who had been a nurse for over thirty years, became her confidante during these nights of panic. When Maya tearfully admitted that she wasn't sure she could handle the responsibility, her aunt's response was blunt but comforting, "if you're this worried about getting it right, that's how I know you're doing it right." It wasn't reassurance so much as permission to stop holding her breath.

The Illusion of Unshakable Authority

The investigation eventually cleared Maya of any wrongdoing, but more importantly, it became a turning point. It did more than confirm her innocence; it exposed the deeper truth behind her fear of failure. Her anxiety about making mistakes was never about her ability to do the job. It came from a perfectionism rooted in the fear that others only saw her as a diversity hire. The real work became shifting that mindset. Rather than fixating on being flawless, she started to see mistakes as part of how she would grow.

She also began to challenge the idea that a leader needed to have all the answers. In a rare moment of honesty, she shared with her team that she did not have everything figured out and that their voices mattered. That moment changed the tone immediately. Nurses who had once been distant started coming to her with questions, ideas, and concerns. They were drawn to a leader who was honest. Someone who showed up fully without pretending to be perfect. For the first time, Maya stopped feeling like she was faking it. She started to feel like a leader. It wasn't because she had all the answers, but because she was committed to finding them together.

As her sense of belonging and support grew, so did her confidence. That confidence gave her the space to reflect and redefine what success actually meant. It was no longer about having it all together. It was about showing up fully, even when it was difficult. That's when she started to let go of the comparison trap. The shift did not happen overnight. It unfolded slowly, in quiet moments. A friend challenged her to write affirmations and stick them to her bathroom mirror. She turned to late-night entries in her journal to debrief from the day and strategize for the next. She made small, yet steady, decisions to keep choosing herself each and every day.

Maya's journey was never about perfection. It was about finding peace in her own voice, her own path, and at her own pace. What once felt like survival slowly became leadership grounded in self trust. She still has hard days, but now she meets them with clarity, not fear. And while the weight never fully disappears, she no longer carries it alone or in silence.

The Role of Career Coaches and Therapists in High Stakes Careers

Maya's story reminds us that imposter syndrome is not just a mindset issue. It is a response to real pressure, real bias, and real fear. But her journey also shows what can shift when you stop carrying it all alone. The kind of breakthrough Maya experienced does not happen in a vacuum. It happens with support. And not just from friends or mentors but through intentional, guided relationships that help you untangle what you have internalized and reframe how you see yourself and your work.

That is where career coaches and therapists come in.

Why You Need Both a Coach and a Therapist

Coaches and therapists do very different work, but together they offer a powerful combination, especially in high pressure careers. A coach focuses on helping you grow professionally. They challenge how you think about leadership, guide your decision making, and give you tools to move strategically in your field. A good coach helps you strengthen your voice, sharpen your goals, and navigate the political realities of your workplace. They help you build confidence that is rooted in performance, not just appearance.

Therapy, on the other hand, is where the deeper work happened for me. Over the course of fifteen years, therapy became the space where I learned how to unpack old beliefs, untangle fear from my identity, and stop confusing survival mechanisms for success strategies. It was the first time I really heard myself think. Without editing. Without performing. That work revealed how much of my drive was actually anxiety, how perfectionism became armor, and how my harsh inner voice sounded a lot like echoes from my past. As we have learned in previous chapters, perfectionism and imposter feelings often reinforce one another, perpetuating the cycle of overachievement and self-doubt.[lxv]

Therapy gave me the tools to slow down long enough to ask myself better questions. It taught me how to challenge thoughts instead of letting them run the show. And it gave me something that coaching alone could not: permission to be a full person, not just a high performer.

Navigating Peer Comparison with a Coach's Guidance

One of the most exhausting parts of imposter syndrome is the mental spiral of comparison. You look around and it seems like everyone else is doing more, moving faster, or making it look easier. That kind of thinking is hard to shut off on your own. A coach helps pull your attention away from what others are doing and redirect it toward your own growth.

Maya's experience mirrors this struggle. She found herself caught in constant comparison, not just to colleagues but to her own mother's legacy. Even as she succeeded, she questioned whether it was enough. "Why doesn't it feel like a win?" she once journaled. "What more do I have to prove?"

I've been there too. I remember scrolling through LinkedIn, seeing updates from peers who seemed so polished and so far ahead. I'd wonder, "am I the only one still trying to catch my breath?" Earlier coaching experiences helped me stop measuring my growth by someone else's highlights. Coaches help you define success based on your values, not just visible wins. They ask questions that challenge you to measure progress in how you handle pressure, how you make decisions, and how you lead with consistency and clarity. When your inner critic tells you that you are falling behind, a coach reminds you to look at the full picture. Growth is not always loud or public. Sometimes the biggest wins are internal.

Addressing Burnout and Building Sustainable Performance

Therapists played a critical role in helping me recognize when burnout was more than just being tired. Over the years, therapy helped me identify the underlying beliefs that kept me overextended. Things like pleasing people, perfectionism, and the need to constantly produce to show my worth to an employer kept me running on my hamster wheel. Chronic burnout is often tied to internalized pressures to achieve and be seen as competent.[lxvi] Therapy gave me the space to examine where those patterns came from and what they were costing me.

I learned how to say "no" without guilt, to rest without shame, and to release the idea that overfunctioning was a badge of honor. I used to wear my exhaustion like proof that I belonged. Now I know better.

Therapy helped me shift from surviving to sustaining, not just in my career, but in my life. Burnout, I came to realize, was the result of carrying too much for too long without allowing myself to set some things down. Therapy taught me to give myself permission to do so.

Owning Expertise Without Overcompensation

Imposter syndrome often tricks high achievers into believing they have to overcompensate. That can look like over preparing, overexplaining, or overthinking. This is all in an attempt to prove you deserve to be in the room. Overcompensation is exhausting as hell, and is not sustainable. It leads to burnout and keeps you stuck in a cycle of trying to earn what you have already proven.

Maya experienced this too. Her attention to detail was relentless, especially during the early pandemic response. One mistake or delay felt like it would confirm every doubt others had about her. That mindset kept her in survival mode.

I recognized that pattern in myself. I used to spend hours perfecting things that were already done just to avoid critique. If it wasn't flawless, it felt like failure. Therapy helped me understand the fear behind that urge. It helped me separate the drive to be excellent from the panic of not being enough.

Coaching helped reinforce that shift by teaching me to reframe what it meant to be an expert. Expertise is not about knowing everything. It is about showing up with clarity, curiosity, and preparation, and having the wisdom

159

to ask questions when needed. True competence includes recognizing what you do not know and still feeling worthy of your role.[lxvii]

Reframing Visibility and Criticism

In high pressure careers, being seen can feel like being exposed. Visibility brings more feedback, more opinions, and more opportunities for criticism. It is easy to become overly cautious or to shrink yourself in response to that kind of attention.

But visibility is not the problem. The fear of what it might expose is. For me, therapy provided the tools to understand where that fear came from. Those old experiences of being judged too harshly, dismissed too quickly, or misunderstood altogether had still been haunting me. I learned to stop internalizing every critique as truth. I stopped viewing every mistake as a threat to my legitimacy.

Coaching played its part by helping me embrace visibility as a sign of growth and impact, not exposure. It reminded me that if people are engaging with your work, even critically, it means they are paying attention. And that matters.

Conclusion: Confidence in High Stakes Careers Is Built, Not Given

Confidence in high pressure environments is not a personality trait you either have or you do not. It is built through reflection, support, and learning to trust yourself even when the doubt creeps in. Coaches and therapists each bring different tools to that process. One helps you move strategically. The other helps you heal deeply. But both are about helping you stand in your own authority with less fear and more clarity.

Imposter syndrome might not disappear overnight. But with the right guidance, it no longer gets to run the show.

PART IV

THRIVING BEYOND IMPOSTER SYNDROME

Chapter 12

Redefining Success on Your Own Terms

Introduction: The Illusion of Success

We're often taught that success is a finish line. That once you hit the right title, land the salary, collect the awards, or finally get your name in rooms that matter, everything else will settle. Your doubt will quiet, your confidence will show up, and life will start making sense. You will believe that you have finally "arrived." But for a lot of high achievers, myself included, it didn't work that way. You reach the goal, and instead of feeling fulfilled, you feel like the clock just reset. The next goal shows up before you even get a chance to breathe. You tell yourself you should feel proud, but all you feel is pressure.

That empty feeling emerges right after the win. It comes from chasing someone else's version of success. We spend so much time proving ourselves with the external stuff such as titles, money, recognition that we forget to ask what actually makes us feel alive, aligned, and whole. The truth is, those outward markers don't mean much if they're disconnected from purpose, passion, or impact. And that's why so many people who look successful on paper still feel lost.

This chapter is about redefining success on your own terms. It's not about giving up on ambition. It's about building a version of success that includes growth, joy, authenticity, and rest, not just performance and pressure. We'll talk about what it looks like to stop climbing for approval and start building a life that actually feels like yours.

The Problem with Society's Definition of Success

The Myth That External Success Creates Confidence

One of the most persistent myths is that external success leads to lasting confidence. This myth assumes that once you achieve a certain status, financial milestone, or level of recognition, self-doubt will vanish. However, confidence that relies primarily on external validation is quite fragile. It can be easily shattered by a single failure, criticism, or competitor's success. The fear of losing what you have achieved or of being exposed as less competent than others becomes overwhelming.

The reason for this fragility is that external success is never truly within your control. It can easily and quickly be stripped away by factors beyond your influence. You are left feeling exposed and unworthy. True confidence, however, is built on the understanding that your worth is not determined by individual outcomes. It is achieved through your resilience, willingness to learn, and ability to adapt. By cultivating this internal form of confidence, you can pursue success without the fear of being exposed, undone, or diminished by failure.

As I am working on this section today I am sitting at a book signing that literally nobody has arrived yet. Am I disappointed, of course. However, I know how many other events have been successful. This poor showing does not shake my confidence. My good friend, Janelle Harper, learned this fully.

Janelle Harper's Story: Breaking Free from the Trap of External Validation

Janelle Harper spent years chasing achievement, believing that each new milestone would silence the self-doubt that followed her throughout her career. Raised in Cleveland, Ohio, she was the first college graduate in her immediate family, earning multiple degrees and quickly advancing in the corporate world. Yet, no matter how many promotions, awards, or accolades she earned, she couldn't shake the feeling that she still had to prove herself.

From an early age, Janelle had associated success with security. Her biological father had been largely absent from her life, and though she had a strong relationship with her stepfather, that early abandonment instilled a deep need to earn validation. She learned to excel academically, to outperform expectations, and to be someone that people couldn't easily overlook.

This mindset followed her into the workplace, where she built an impressive career in recruitment, compliance, and diversity, equity, and inclusion. She was known as a leader in her field, developing policies that helped shape company culture and winning national DEI awards for her work. Still, imposter syndrome clung to her, reinforced by

165

the unspoken but ever-present reality of being a Black woman in corporate America.

Even when she sat at leadership tables, she often felt like an outsider. She noticed that while her expertise was respected in theory, she wasn't always included in the decisions that truly mattered. Her work was praised, until it challenged the status quo. Her input was valued, until it became inconvenient. When leadership changes occurred, she was reminded that no matter how much she had contributed, she was not seen as one of them.

Perfectionism and Overcompensation: The Exhausting Chase for Approval

To counteract these challenges, Janelle overprepared for every meeting, pursued extra certifications, and took on more work than necessary. She feared that any misstep would confirm the doubts she had about herself. Worse, she would confirm the negative assumptions others had about her. Perfectionism became a shield, a way to feel in control in an environment where Black women are often scrutinized more harshly, expected to be twice as good just to be seen as competent.

Yet, the more she achieved, the higher the stakes became. Success didn't bring confidence. It brought a new level of pressure. She felt like she couldn't afford to fail, because failure wasn't just personal. It was proof that she never belonged in the first place.

This is the trap of external validation. When confidence is tied to achievement, there is no finish line. Every success only sets the bar higher, leaving no space to pause and acknowledge progress. For Janelle, each new accomplishment only fueled a cycle of chasing, proving, and exhausting herself in the process.

The Breaking Point: Realizing External Success Would Never Be Enough

Janelle's realization came when, despite all she had done to transform her company's DEI efforts, she was overlooked when it truly mattered. She had led initiatives that changed company culture, secured funding for major programs, and positioned the company as a national leader in DEI. Yet, when it came time for key leadership decisions, she was still excluded from the inner circle.

It was a painful but eye-opening moment. She had done everything right. She had performed at the highest level. But at the end of the day, no amount of external success could change a system that was never fully built to include her.

For the first time, she questioned whether she was climbing the right ladder. Had she been chasing success in an environment where she would never truly feel valued?

Redefining Confidence on Her Own Terms

Janelle eventually left corporate America to start her own consulting firm. The decision wasn't easy. Walking away from a structured career meant leaving behind the traditional markers of success she had relied on for validation. She worried that no one would take her seriously without a company attached to her name.

But stepping into entrepreneurship forced her to do something she had never done before She defined success for herself.

For the first time, she wasn't waiting for a corporation to tell her she was good enough. She wasn't seeking leadership's approval or trying to fit into a space that was reluctant to fully embrace her. She was owning her expertise, her voice, and her worth. She was not waiting for anyone's permission but her own.

Now, Janelle mentors emerging leaders, helping them recognize their value before they spend years proving it to others. She teaches women and professionals of color how to redefine confidence as something built internally, rather than something granted externally.

Though self-doubt still appears from time to time, she has learned that imposter syndrome is not a reflection of her ability. It is a byproduct of a system that was never designed for her success. Instead of proving herself to others, she focuses on building the kind of success that feels meaningful to her.

The Lesson: Confidence Comes from Within, Not From Validation

Janelle's story is a clear example of how external success does not cure imposter syndrome. Confidence built on validation is fleeting. It is easily shaken by exclusion, bias, or shifting workplace dynamics. When your sense of worth is tied to achievement, the goalpost will always move.

True confidence is not about waiting for others to recognize your success. Rather, it is about recognizing it yourself. It means understanding that your value is not determined by a job title, a promotion, or a seat at someone else's table.

By separating identity from external success, you free yourself from the exhausting cycle of proving and chasing. Instead of asking, *do they see me as successful?* you begin to ask, *do I feel fulfilled?* And in answering that question, you take back control of your own confidence.

The Hollow Victory Phenomenon

Hollow victories happen when the accomplishments you work so hard for don't actually meet your deeper needs, such as purpose, connection, or a sense of fulfillment. This experience is especially common among high achievers who spend most of their energy chasing external symbols of success such as titles, income, or recognition. They chase these symbols without pausing to ask if those goals align with their values or passions. Reaching each new milestone brings a short burst of relief but rarely delivers lasting satisfaction.[lxviii]

Hollow victories hit differently. They feel "empty" because they're not connected to what really drives us deep down, like learning, making a difference, or just keeping real with ourselves. When achievements are pursued for the sake of appearance or to prove worth to others they cannot fulfill the deeper needs for meaning and alignment. The internal question remains unanswered, "*am I doing what truly matters to me?*"

I've chased quite a few of those wins before. If I am being honest, I still do, albeit much less. The titles, applause, even a bigger paycheck are still real things for me, just like all of us human beings. They look great on paper, in the driveway or in the bank account. But when the dust settles, I have been left with some pyrrhic victories. Something was still missing. That's when I realized that it's not just about what you accomplish. What truly matters is whether it actually means something to you.

Escaping the cycle of hollow victories requires redefining success based on what genuinely brings you joy, growth, and a sense of purpose. This involves turning inward to assess what matters most to you—beyond what is impressive to others or recognized by society.

The Role of Passion and Purpose in Redefining Success

While the terms "passion" and "purpose" are often used interchangeably, they serve distinct roles in defining a meaningful version of success. Passion is about what excites and energizes you. The activities that make time disappear because you are so deeply engaged. Passion is often linked to the things you enjoy doing for their own sake, without any external reward. Purpose, on the other hand, is about the impact you want to have. The broader significance of your actions beyond personal gratification. Purpose is rooted in serving something larger than

170

yourself, whether that's your community, your industry, or a cause you care about.

I am passionate about the work that I do in my 9-5. It is important to me to support the team I oversee as they help the citizens of the City of Cleveland. Conversely, I feel that I am living further in my purpose in the work I accomplish in my 5-9. Being a consultant to small business and nonprofits, mentoring students, and writing and presenting on topics such as imposter syndrome, leadership, and communication are in line with that purpose.

Aligning your definition of success with both passion and purpose transforms it from a relentless chase into a fulfilling journey. When you pursue goals that reflect your passions, you find joy in the process itself. When those goals also serve your sense of purpose, they bring a deeper form of satisfaction. External trappings cannot provide that level of fulfillment alone. This dual alignment makes success sustainable, meaningful, and immune to the fleeting nature of external validation.

James Holloway's journey is a testament to this transformation.

From Proving Himself to Finding Purpose

Growing up in the Lee and Harvard area of Cleveland, Ohio, James Holloway didn't have many professional role models. The people around him worked hard, but few had access to higher education or corporate careers. He was bright and ambitious, but without guidance, he struggled to envision what success could look like beyond survival.

There were no mentors to show him the way, no blueprint for building a career in finance, and no professionals in his community who could validate his aspirations.

James was the first in his immediate family to attend college, and without a clear sense of direction, he latched onto one belief. To succeed, he had to be better. He needed to be twice as good, twice as qualified, and twice as credentialed. He pursued higher education relentlessly, earning five degrees, including an MBA and multiple certifications in accounting and finance. At every milestone, he felt temporary relief, but soon the self-doubt would creep back in. *What if I don't actually know enough? What if I'm missing something critical?*

James' imposter syndrome was a vicious cycle. The belief that he needed just one more credential before he could feel secure defined the early years of his career. But something changed when he joined his accounting firm.

James currently serves as a project manager at the firm, overseeing financial operations and managing critical projects. However, his passion for inclusion and mentorship led him to take on collateral duties outside of his primary role. Recognizing the challenges faced by underrepresented professionals in corporate spaces, he spearheaded the firm's diversity, equity, and inclusion (DEI) initiatives. He didn't take this on because it was required, but because he believed in making a difference.

Instead of feeling like just another employee, James found an environment that valued his perspective. His firm supported his vision when he took the lead on these initiatives, allowing him to create programs that fostered inclusion within the company. Suddenly, his work wasn't just about financial statements and compliance. It was about shaping the culture of the firm and ensuring that future generations of professionals wouldn't feel as isolated as he once did, especially those from underrepresented backgrounds.

Leading the firm's DEI efforts gave James something that all his credentials never could. A sense of purpose. He saw the real impact of his efforts. Mentoring young professionals, opening doors for others, and advocating for international DEI initiatives that would reshape the industry became his purpose. His focus shifted from proving himself to empowering others.

Outside of work, James now dedicates his time to mentoring students in STEM fields. He is providing the kind of guidance he wished he had growing up. He helps young people from similar backgrounds see that they don't need to overcompensate with endless credentials to belong in professional spaces. They just need the confidence to step into them.

For years, James thought success was about doing more. He needed more degrees, more certifications, and more achievements. Now, he understands that true success is about doing what matters. His passion for finance remains, but his purpose is in making sure the next generation of professionals can walk into the rooms he once felt unworthy of with their heads held high.

The Trap of Moving Goalposts

The "moving goalpost" mindset keeps high achievers stuck in a loop where nothing ever feels like enough. The moment they hit a goal, the bar shifts. They tell themselves it wasn't that big of a deal or that it came too easily, so they set a new, harder one. Underneath it all is a fear that if they pause to celebrate, they'll get too comfortable. Or, heaven forbid, people will realize their success was just luck.

For those with imposter syndrome, especially those who fall into the expert subtype, this cycle can be relentless. The belief that one more degree, one more certification or leadership role will finally bring confidence, only leads to temporary relief, not true fulfillment. Instead of internalizing success, high achievers in this cycle constantly raise the bar, believing they need to accomplish more before they can feel worthy.

Simone Whitfield-Hayes knows this cycle all too well.

Simone's Story: The Credentials Were Never Enough

Simone Whitfield-Hayes has spent her entire career chasing the next credential, believing that success was something she had to earn over and over again. As a vice president at a national nonprofit, she holds degrees in engineering and law, has led multi-million-dollar initiatives, and is widely respected in her field. Yet, despite all of this, she still wonders whether she is truly qualified.

As the first college graduate in her immediate family, Simone felt an immense responsibility to succeed. This pressure was increased by the need to be successful for the people who had supported her even more than for herself. Growing up in Detroit, she was labeled the smart girl early on. Teachers placed her in advanced classes, and expectations were set for her success before she even had the chance to define what success meant for herself. She excelled in math and science, which naturally led her to engineering. But in college, as one of the few Black women in her program, she became hyper-aware of how often she had to prove herself in ways her peers did not. While other students seemed to move forward with confidence, she constantly second-guessed whether she was as competent as she appeared.

During her undergraduate years, Simone joined a prominent sorority within the "Divine Nine," an experience that gave her a deep sense of sisterhood and community. She quickly became active in leadership, holding multiple positions both as a student and later a graduate member. Her involvement in the sorority strengthened her networking skills and gave her opportunities to lead outside of the workplace, but even within that space, she often felt the need to prove herself. While she was respected, she sometimes wondered if she was truly making an impact or if she was simply "checking the boxes" of leadership.

After earning her engineering degree, Simone made a pivot into law, believing that a legal career would offer even more stability. Yet, even after passing the bar exam,

175

she didn't feel ready to practice. Instead of recognizing her expertise, she convinced herself that she needed more experience, more training, something more before she could truly own the title of lawyer.

Her self-doubt was compounded by the pressures of balancing her career with motherhood. As a mother of two, she often felt torn between professional ambition and the expectation to be fully present for her children. No matter how much she accomplished, she couldn't shake the feeling that she wasn't doing enough in either role.

This mindset followed her into leadership. When she was encouraged to apply for a senior executive position, her first instinct was doubt. *Am I really ready for this? Is there someone more qualified?* Despite already managing teams, leading projects, and making critical decisions, she believed she lacked something. This belief was reinforced by years of measuring her worth against an ever-moving standard of enough.

The reality was, Simone had already proven herself countless times, but she had never stopped to recognize it. Instead, she had fallen into the moving goalpost trap where every milestone she reached immediately became the new minimum expectation.

Breaking the Cycle of Perpetual Achievement

Simone's story is far from unique. Many professionals, particularly women and people of color, feel an unspoken pressure to continually prove their worth through achievements. Their success is often seen as conditional.

They are validated only if they continue to excel at increasingly higher levels.

Escaping this trap involves practicing the skill of acknowledgment. It requires pausing to reflect on and internalize achievements before moving on to the next goal. This doesn't mean abandoning ambition, but rather balancing it with appreciation for what has already been accomplished.

Simone is still learning this. Instead of chasing another certification or degree, she is working on recognizing that her success is not something she has to keep re-earning. The truth is, she was qualified long before she believed she was.

For anyone caught in the trap of moving goalposts, the real challenge is not in achieving more. To be clear, their true challenge is in learning to finally accept that they are already enough.

Success as a Daily Practice

Success is not a distant destination. It is a series of daily actions and choices that align with your values and passions. Success should be treated as something you do, not something you achieve. This transforms it from an outcome you chase, to something you do innately. This approach makes success accessible every day, not just at the culmination of a major goal.

This practice-oriented mindset involves consciously making decisions that reflect your values, celebrating small wins along the way, and embracing progress rather than perfection. When success becomes a habit rather than a horizon, it is easier to feel fulfilled and confident, even in the midst of pursuing bigger goals.

Reframing Failure Through Self-Compassion

Real success means rethinking what failure actually is. It's not a statement about your value. It is just a part of the process of growing. When you give yourself some grace and stop beating yourself up, failure stops being something to hide from and starts becoming something you learn from. That kind of self-compassion gives you the courage to take risks, mess up, and still get back up and keep pushing forward.

When you can view failure as feedback rather than a flaw, you free yourself to experiment, learn, and evolve without the paralyzing fear of being exposed as inadequate. This shift allows you to pursue success with a growth mindset. Your focus shifts to learning and adapting rather than protecting your self-image.

Conclusion: Success Is a Journey, Not a Destination

True success is about alignment with your values, pursuit of meaningful goals, and the ability to find joy in the journey rather than in the destination. When success is defined by growth, impact, passion, and fulfillment, it becomes a source of energy and motivation rather than a cause of burnout. By redefining success on your own terms, you reclaim the power to shape a life that is both successful and deeply satisfying.

Chapter 13

When Your Past Haunts Your Potential

Reclaiming Identity After Success

Imposter syndrome is primarily discussed as something that surfaces on the upward climb toward achievement. It manifests as you build your reputation or find space in unfamiliar professional environments. But what's less explored, and perhaps more crafty, is the version that emerges after the climb. After you have your career-defining moment and milestone(s). After the accolades have faded into memory and routine replaces applause.

This version doesn't whisper that you never belonged. Instead, it tells you that you did, but no longer do. It lives in the gap between who you were and who you are now, casting a shadow over everything you try to become next. It's not driven by fear of being discovered as a fraud. It's driven by fear that your most valuable self already came and went. All that now remains is the obligation to preserve the image.

This is Has-Been Syndrome.

What Is Has-Been Syndrome?

Has-Been Syndrome is a lesser-known form of imposter syndrome rooted not in self-doubt about potential, but in grief over a version of self that once commanded attention, respect, and certainty. It is most common in those who have experienced early success, high visibility, or strong identity attachment to a specific role or title. This syndrome doesn't ask, "*Am I enough?*" It declares, "*I was once, but I don't know if I still am.*"

Rather than questioning their initial achievements, those grappling with Has-Been Syndrome question whether they have anything left to offer beyond them. They may find themselves recounting past accolades more than exploring new aspirations. They turn down unfamiliar opportunities out of fear they might not measure up. Or they compare their current reality to the height of their former self. It is not the absence of confidence, but the absence of clarity after a role has ended. Voluntarily or otherwise.

The danger of Has-Been Syndrome lies not in nostalgia itself, but in the way it transforms your identity. The past becomes not just a place to visit, but a place to live. And in doing so, the future becomes less about possibility and more about preservation.

The Psychology of Has-Been Syndrome

Has-Been Syndrome is not a simple reaction to change. It is the result of several deeper psychological and emotional dynamics converging at once. It becomes a culmination of identity disruption, ego attachment, and cultural myths about where worth comes from and when it ends.

Identity Disruption

Eventually, most people shift from being asked, "What do you do?" to defining themselves by who they are. The lines blur between function and identity, role and worth. The doctor becomes the healer. The litigator becomes the fighter. The founder becomes the visionary. Over time, we stop distinguishing between what we contribute and who we are. The loss of that contribution feels like you have lost yourself.

When those roles disappear—whether through retirement, transition, layoff, or personal choice—it's not just a shift in job description. It's a rupture in identity. For high achievers especially, the sense of self-worth is so deeply tied to performance that any change feels like failure, even when it's not. This is not a loss of title but a loss of orientation. Without the familiar structure of our past identity, we lose the mirror that once confirmed our significance.

Ego and Nostalgia

The ego, often misunderstood as arrogance, is in many ways a defense mechanism. It is the internal guardian of status, visibility, and perceived value. When faced with uncertainty, it retreats into certainty. And certainty, for those haunted by their former success, often lives in the past.

Nostalgia becomes the balm. A way to feel powerful again, even if only in memory. But when nostalgia is not balanced by vision, it becomes a trap. What begins as pride in what once was slowly morphs into avoidance of what could be. We repackage stories from our prime, retell them to new audiences, and construct identity around memories rather than current movement. This is not vanity. It is a fear that who we once were is the best we will ever be.

The Myth of the Peak

Our culture glorifies the idea of peaking. You have reached your professional or personal high point early in your career. You peaked! Now you spend the rest of life trying to maintain, replicate, or mourn it. Entire industries (entertainment, fashion, sports, etc.) profit from the notion that youth, early achievement, and first breakthroughs define one's value. By contrast, later-life reinvention is rarely celebrated unless it mimics earlier forms of success.

This myth teaches people that their greatest contributions must occur in a fixed window of time, and that anything after that window is a lesser version of themselves. But purpose does not age out. Creativity does not expire. Wisdom often arrives when the noise fades, not when the crowd cheers.

Still, when Has-Been Syndrome takes root, the myth of the peak feels like the truth. And it convinces even the most accomplished people that their value lives behind them.

The Cost of Staying Stuck

Holding on too tightly to who you used to be might feel comfortable, but eventually it starts to wear you down. That old version of you stops being a foundation to build on and becomes a ceiling that you're stuck on. Instead of stretching into new possibilities, you end up shrinking to fit into outdated ones.

Professionally, that might look like turning down opportunities that push you, just to stay in familiar territory. Emotionally, it can show up as bitterness, isolation, or quietly resenting others who've evolved. Financially, you might find yourself overspending just to uphold an old image. And relationally, it creates distance, especially from those who connect with the person you're becoming, not the one you're clinging to.

Maybe the most harmful part of staying stuck isn't what happens on the outside. It's what happens inside. Your curiosity fades. You stop wondering what's possible, and in that stillness, you stop growing. You slip into survival mode, replaying old stories and avoiding new moves out of fear they'll expose how much you've slipped.

But here's the truth: staying in the same place doesn't preserve who you are. It only delays who you're meant to become.

Reclaiming the Future: The Five Steps to Healing Has-Been Syndrome

Grieve the Old You

The first step in healing Has-Been Syndrome is not reinvention. It's the release. Reinvention without grief is just substitution. Until you acknowledge what has ended, you will always carry it with you. Silently comparing your next chapter to a story that's already closed.

Letting go of who you used to be isn't easy; but it's necessary. And honestly, it's a sign of self-respect. You're not turning your back on your past, you're just acknowledging that it had its time. Maybe that looks like journaling, thinking back on old wins and losses, or just sitting in that weird in-between space where you're not who you were, but not quite who you're becoming either. It's uncomfortable but if you don't take the time to grieve that old identity, you'll keep dragging it with you. And that weight holds you back from fully stepping into who you're meant to be next.

Remember Al Bundy from *Married with Children*? His greatest point in life was the "four touchdowns he scored in a single game at Polk High." He never moved beyond that peak. In fact, he ended every evening, hands resting in his waistband and resting on his couch and telling anyone (or himself) about those four touchdowns.

Redefine Success in This Season

One of the reasons Has-Been Syndrome lingers is because we cling to outdated definitions of success. When those definitions no longer align with our present lives, we assume something is wrong with us, rather than with the measure.

Success evolves. What once meant status may now mean stability. What once centered on recognition may now center on relevance or service. Reclaiming your life means allowing your values to lead. Not your résumé.

Ask yourself, "what does success look like now?" Is it the same as what it used to look like? Name what matters to you. Identify what gives you energy. Let this be the season where success is defined not by what impresses others, but by what sustains you.

Become a Beginner Again

Perhaps the most frightening and most necessary part of healing from Has-Been Syndrome is the willingness to be new again. To enter spaces where you don't have all the answers. To be taught. To fail. To not be impressive, but present.

For high achievers, the idea of starting over can feel humbling, or worse, humiliating. It's the guts to start over that gets things moving again. That first brave step sparks the momentum you've been missing. Let go of the need to master skills immediately. Embrace the awkwardness of being a neophyte again. Honor the learning curve. This is not a fall from grace, it is a return to growth.

Stop Performing, Start Building

There's a big difference between showing up and showing off. One comes from being fully present. The other is about holding on...trying to preserve an image. If you catch yourself performing a version of you that doesn't feel real anymore, that's your signal. Time to drop the mask.

Rebuilding doesn't usually happen in the spotlight. It starts in the small, quiet moments. It's not when you take on things to impress or gain accolades. It is because something real was stirred in you. And yeah, building takes more time than performing. What you actually build far outlasts the applause.

Tell a New Story About Yourself

The final step in reclaiming your identity is rewriting your narrative. You are not obligated to introduce yourself by your former title, or to frame your story around your most celebrated season. You have permission to speak from where you are. Not where you were.

Craft a new introduction that reflects your values, not your résumé. Practice naming what you are building rather than what you have lost. Let your story reflect who you are becoming. Not just who you used to be.

You're Not a Has-Been. You're Becoming.

Has-Been Syndrome is not a death sentence. It is a signal that something inside you is ready to change. That the past has been honored. But not at the cost of your future.

You are still capable and creative. You're called to contribute.

This chapter of your life may not be about applause, but it can be quite peaceful. Allow (or force) yourself to evolve. This is not because your former self was a failure, but because you are still growing.

That is what becoming is all about, as T.J. eventually figured out.

A Glimpse of Glory

The lights were brightest on Friday nights in Jacksonville, North Carolina. Terrance "T.J." DeShields could feel them—not just on his skin, but in his chest. He was eighteen and electrifying. The town turned out to see him run, hit, lead. He had the kind of early promise that demanded attention. By twenty-one, he was shaking hands with NFL executives. By twenty-five, no one was returning his calls.

T.J. had lived the dream, even if only for a moment. Drafted, traded, injured, and quietly let go. There was no headline marking the end. No public announcement. Just a slow fade. The loss wasn't loud, it was internal. And perhaps more devastating for that very reason. What followed wasn't a collapse, but a performance. T.J. wasn't chasing a future, he was holding onto his old identity.

The Illusion of Still Being "That Guy"

After the league, he moved through the world with a certain practiced confidence. He maintained a firm handshake, polished look, and a story always queued up about "back when I was in the league." He drove leased cars, wore designer clothes he could barely afford, and made appearances in places where people still remembered who he was. But it was all a performance.

In private, he was exhausted. He turned down job offers that didn't match the image. Avoided spaces where he'd be unknown or, worse, unimpressive. His world got smaller, but his stories got louder. He wasn't growing. He was clinging to his identity that no longer matched his reality.

What he feared most wasn't obscurity. It was feeling irrelevant.

The Question That Changed Everything

It wasn't until a quiet Thanksgiving morning that something cracked open. T.J. had flown home, hungover from a long night out, still playing the part. His father—a retired Marine, methodical and measured—was outside raking leaves.

"Grab that other rake," he said.

They worked in silence for a while. Then his father stopped.

"You remember who you were before they started calling your name?"

T.J. looked down. "Not really."

"I do," his father said. "You were curious. Thoughtful. Used to build things. You had a mind before you had muscle. The league didn't make you. It just borrowed you."

Then came the sentence that stayed with him.

"Don't die holdin' onto that chapter son."

The Long Work of Becoming

That conversation didn't lead to a grand reinvention. There was no media profile, no dramatic pivot. Just small, humbling steps. He returned to college. Sat quietly in the back of classrooms surrounded by students a decade younger. Group projects made him uneasy. He didn't like being "just a student." But he kept going.

Eventually, he took an unpaid internship at a real estate development firm. Filed papers. Ran errands. Sat in meetings where no one cared who he used to be. It stung at first. Over time he realized something important; he wasn't pretending anymore. He was learning, building, and becoming.

He studied the real estate and investment markets. Learned the streets. He began seeing neighborhoods differently. They were communities. He started negotiating small deals. Then bigger ones. And slowly, the confidence that once came from a jersey began to come from something deeper.

A New Story

There came a point where he stopped introducing himself as a former NFL player. Not because he was ashamed, but because it no longer defined him.

"My name is Terrance DeShields," he began saying. "I build futures."

That was it. Not a title. Not a highlight reel. Just purpose.

And at that moment, he took the pen back. Not to rewrite the past, but to author the future.

Chapter 14

You Belong at the Table—Now What

et's keep it real. Reaching "the table" is a beautiful, earned moment. But it's also where imposter syndrome gets real pervasive.

> *Hey you. Good morning. Today might be the day. Man, I hope they do not actually pay attention to your presentation because they will finally see you for who you really are. Yikes, Oh well, it was fun while it lasted though, right?*

It constantly taps you on your shoulder. It doesn't leave the room once you arrive, it changes its disguise. Now the voice says *"okay, you're here...but for how long?"* Or, *"you made it, but can you really keep up?"*

I've felt that. Despite becoming published, giving a keynote, or being honored, there are days I still look around a room and wonder if someone's about to call me out. Not because I've done something wrong, but because that old tape in my head tries to convince me I somehow finessed my way in.

That's the thing about imposter syndrome. It does not give a damn about your résumé. It doesn't care how many people clap for you. It cares about whether you've internalized your worth.

From Surviving to Owning It

Here's the hard truth, overcoming imposter syndrome isn't just about affirmations or career milestones. It's about rewiring how you were built to think. Many of us didn't just wake up with self-doubt. We were conditioned into it by trauma, by marginalization, by systems that made us earn every inch of our progress. It's not just our inner critic that we're up against. It's our wiring.

Some of us were raised in survival mode. We didn't learn confidence. We learned fear and caution. We didn't grow up hearing "you belong here," We heard, "don't mess this up." So even when we win, we brace for loss. That's what makes imposter syndrome so hard to shake. It isn't just fear. It's familiar.

Let's go back to some of the folks we met along the way.

Malcolm, for instance. The one who could command a room with his presence but couldn't quiet the inner doubt whispering that he was one mistake away from being exposed. His journey wasn't about finding more confidence. It was about unlearning the belief that visibility and vulnerability were threats.

Or Izzy. Man, she fought hard. Bar exam, ADHD, financial pressure, all of it. But she learned something so powerful. You don't wait until the doubt disappears to show up. You show up *despite* it. Her wiring was forged in scarcity and perfectionism, but she still made room for grace. Each time she cracked a book again, each affirmation she wrote, she wasn't just studying. She was pushing back against every inherited voice that told her she wasn't enough.

Or take Julissa. Her story sits at the intersection of so many identities—immigrant, woman, mother, aspiring attorney. The world has told her in a thousand ways she doesn't belong. But she's still pushing forward. That's tenacity. That's resilience. She's not just moving through imposter syndrome; she's dragging entire legacies of silence and invisibility with her and saying, "No more."

Then there's T.J., who spent years clinging to an identity that no longer fit because he didn't believe the new version of himself was worthy without the applause. He wasn't rebuilding a career. He was rebuilding self-worth. That's the deeper work. That's what this chapter of his life is all about.

And me? I've lived this book. I've sat across from partners in a law firm wondering if they saw the lawyer, the marine, the East Clevelander or, heaven forbid, the stripper. I've delivered keynotes with a smile on my face and a pit in my stomach. I've earned degrees and titles, but still wake up some mornings waiting for the shoe to drop. The hardest work I've done isn't in business or law. It has been battling the narrative that I'm somehow a fluke. A fake. Convincing and reminding myself that I am the result of learning and following my plan for success looks like. Not a lucky break or two.

Before we wrap up, let's talk about what all of this means in practice. When you've carried self-doubt for years, it can be hard to even know what confidence really looks like. And yet, the next level in this journey is not just surviving imposter syndrome. It's learning how to lead through it. That's the work now. Show up with truth, with courage, and with integrity in the face of that inner friction.

What It Means to Lead Authentically

Let's also be clear, leadership isn't just about how you manage a team or navigate your career. It's about how you manage yourself. How you steady your mind when it starts spinning. How you talk to yourself after a mistake. How you choose to show up when you'd rather shrink. Authentic leadership begins within. It's self-awareness in action. It's making decisions not out of fear, but from clarity and conviction.

True leadership isn't about having all the answers. It's about being willing to ask the right questions! It's about staying teachable, coachable, and grounded. Not perfect, but present.

Confidence doesn't mean the absence of fear. It means you trust yourself enough to keep showing up anyway. Especially when your own thoughts try to sabotage you.

When I started I.S.I. Consulting, I didn't have a blueprint. Just a belief that maybe my mistakes could be someone else's shortcut. That belief is what led me to this book, these stories, and these lessons.

So no, you don't have to pretend to have it all together. What you do have to do is keep building the muscle of self-trust. That's what Layla did. She didn't let her humility keep her invisible. She allowed herself to own her impact without apology. Not with arrogance, but with clarity.

Your Turn to Reclaim the Narrative

By now, I hope you see that imposter syndrome isn't some character flaw to fix. It's a signal. A nudge. A reminder that you care, that you're growing, that you've stepped outside of your comfort zone. And yes, it's also a scar. One that tells a story of the fights you've survived. You have fought valiantly against systems, against expectations, and sometimes against yourself.

But here's the truth. You belong at the table *because* of what you've been through. Because of the resilience you've shown. Because of the fire that still burns even when the path ahead isn't clear.

And if you've got a voice in your head asking, "*Who do you think you are?,*" then answer it.

> *Say, "I'm someone who's done the work. I'm someone who isn't faking it. I am figuring out the game and looking good as I do it." Say, "I belong here. I earned this. And I'm getting better everyday".*

The table's not just lucky to have you. It needs you.

See you there.

FINAL THOUGHTS

If this book spoke to you—if it helped you feel seen, validated, or just a little less alone in your struggle with imposter syndrome—I'd be grateful if you'd leave a quick review on Amazon.

Your review doesn't have to be long or fancy. Just honest. Reviews help other readers (especially the ones still doubting themselves) decide to take a chance on a book that might be exactly what they need.

And if you're looking for more real-world tools and guidance, check out my first book *Unlocking Potential: Insights, Tips & Strategies for Young Black Professionals*, along with its companion workbook. Both are available on Amazon, Barnes and Noble (online) or at www.isiconsultingllc.com.

Thank you for reading *Overcoming Imposter Syndrome: You Belong at the Table*. And thank you for being proof that we can do hard things—and still be vulnerable enough to tell the truth about them.

Tony

ABOUT THE AUTHOR

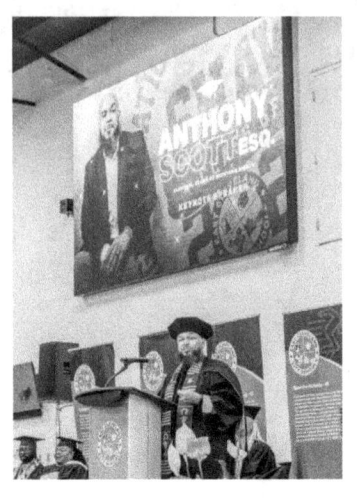

Anthony (Tony) W. Scott, Esq. has decades of leadership and management experience drawn from a wide-ranging career in private industry, public interest, government, and entrepreneurship. His leadership journey began with his service in the United States Marine Corps during Operations Desert Storm and Desert Shield. A first-generation college graduate, Tony went on to earn a Master's Degree in Public Administration and a Juris Doctorate.

Tony is also the author of *Unlocking Potential: Insights, Tips & Strategies for Young Black Professionals*, a practical guidebook rooted in real-life experience and designed to inspire the next generation of leaders. That book, and its companion workbook, reflect the same core philosophy that defines all of Tony's work: transparency, authenticity, and a commitment to lifting others as he climbs.

A true open book, Tony candidly shares the missteps and lessons he's learned so others can avoid the same pitfalls. This commitment to "not hiding the ball" led him to create I.S.I. Consulting, LLC, where he lives by the mantra: *Build Solutions Today, Avoid Pitfalls Tomorrow.*

To learn more or schedule a speaking engagement, visit www.isiconsultingllc.com or email Tony directly at info@isiconsultingllc.com.

NOTES

[i] This quote is widely attributed to Maya Angelou and frequently appears in literature and media discussing imposter syndrome, though the original source (book, interview, or speech) has not been definitively documented. See: Goodreads. (n.d.). *Quote by Maya Angelou.* Retrieved from https://www.goodreads.com/quotes/220406

[ii] Holt, J. (2005, February 28). *Time Bandits: What Were Einstein and Gödel Talking About?* The New Yorker. Retrieved from https://www.newyorker.com/magazine/2005/02/28/time-bandits-2

[iii] Beck, A. T. (1976). *Cognitive Therapy and the Emotional Disorders.* New York: International Universities Press.

[iv] Kruger, J., & Dunning, D. (1999). *Unskilled and unaware of it: How difficulties in recognizing one's own incompetence lead to inflated self-assessments.* Journal of Personality and Social Psychology, 77(6), 1121–1134. https://doi.org/10.1037/0022-3514.77.6.1121

[v] Kruger (1999), 1121–1134.

[vi] Festinger, L. (1957). *A Theory of Cognitive Dissonance.* Stanford University Press.

[vii] Brown, B. (2010). *The Gifts of Imperfection: Let Go of Who You Think You're Supposed to Be and Embrace Who You Are.* Hazelden Publishing.

[viii] Flett, G. L., & Hewitt, P. L. (2002). *Perfectionism: Theory, Research, and Treatment.* American Psychological Association.

[ix] Clance, P. R., & Imes, S. A. (1978). *The Impostor Phenomenon in High Achieving Women: Dynamics and Therapeutic Intervention.* Psychotherapy: Theory, Research & Practice, 15(3), 241–247. https://doi.org/10.1037/h0086006

[x] Frost, R. O., Marten, P., Lahart, C., & Rosenblate, R. (1990). *The dimensions of perfectionism. Cognitive Therapy and Research*, 14(5), 449–468. https://doi.org/10.1007/BF01172967

[xi] Aaron T. Beck, *Cognitive Therapy and the Emotional Disorders* (New York: International Universities Press, 1976); David D. Burns, *The Feeling Good Handbook* (New York: Plume, 1989).

[xii] Stoeber, J., & Damian, L. E. (2016). *Perfectionism in employees: Work engagement, workaholism, and burnout*. In Flett, G. L., & Hewitt, P. L. (Eds.), *Perfectionism: A relational approach to conceptualization, assessment, and treatment* (pp. 265–283). American Psychological Association. https://doi.org/10.1037/14861-013

[xiii] Beck, A. T., & Emery, G. (1985). *Anxiety Disorders and Phobias: A Cognitive Perspective*. Basic Books.

[xiv] For foundational research on attributional styles and success attribution bias, see: Bernard Weiner, *Judgments of Responsibility: A Foundation for a Theory of Social Conduct* (New York: Guilford Press, 1995). See also Clance (1978) 241–247.

[xv] U.S. Dept. of Housing and Urban Development.

[xvi] Young, V. (2011). *The Secret Thoughts of Successful Women: Why Capable People Suffer from the Impostor Syndrome and How to Thrive in Spite of It*. Crown Business.

[xvii] American Psychological Association. (2023). *Ethnic and Racial Disparities: Key Definitions – Implicit Bias*. https://www.apa.org/topics/racism-bias-discrimination/types

[xviii] McCluney, C. L., Robotham, K., Lee, S., Smith, R., & Durkee, M. (2019). The costs of code-switching. *Harvard Business Review*. https://hbr.org/2019/11/the-costs-of-codeswitching

[xix] Jamieson, K. H. (1995). *Beyond the Double Bind: Women and Leadership*. Oxford University Press.

[xx] Clance (1978), 241–247.

[xxi] Young (2011).

[xxii] Tokenism is when an organization includes a small number of people from underrepresented groups just to look diverse, without giving them real power or support. These individuals often feel isolated and pressured to represent their entire group. Catalyst. (2021). *Tokenism.* Retrieved from https://www.catalyst.org/research/tokenism/

[xxiii] Cisgender refers to a person whose gender identity aligns with the sex they were assigned at birth. For example, someone who was assigned female at birth and identifies as a woman is considered cisgender. American Psychological Association. (2015). *Guidelines for Psychological Practice with Transgender and Gender Nonconforming People.* https://www.apa.org/practice/guidelines/transgender.pdf

[xxiv] McKinsey & Company. (2020). *How the LGBTQ+ community fares in the workplace.* Retrieved from https://www.mckinsey.com/featured-insights/diversity-and-inclusion/how-the-lgbtq-plus-community-fares-in-the-workplace

[xxv] LeDoux, J. E. (1996). *The Emotional Brain: The Mysterious Underpinnings of Emotional Life.* Simon & Schuster.

[xxvi] Lieberman, M. D. (2013). *Social: Why Our Brains Are Wired to Connect.* Crown Publishers.

[xxvii] LeDoux, J. (2015). *Anxious: Using the Brain to Understand and Treat Fear and Anxiety.* Viking.

[xxviii] Kross, E., & Ayduk, Ö. (2011). Making meaning out of negative experiences by self-distancing. *Current Directions in Psychological Science*, 20(3), 187–191.

[xxix] LeDoux, J. E. (2000). *Emotion circuits in the brain.* Annual Review of Neuroscience, 23(1), 155–184. https://doi.org/10.1146/annurev.neuro.23.1.155

[xxx] Phelps, E. A., & LeDoux, J. E. (2005). *Contributions of the amygdala to emotion processing: From animal models to human behavior.* Neuron, 48(2), 175–187. https://doi.org/10.1016/j.neuron.2005.09.025

[xxxi]Ohman, A., & Mineka, S. (2001). *Fears, phobias, and preparedness: Toward an evolved module of fear and fear learning*. Psychological Review, 108(3), 483–522. https://doi.org/10.1037/0033-295X.108.3.483

[xxxii] Sapolsky, R. M. (2017). *Behave: The Biology of Humans at Our Best and Worst*. Penguin Press.

[xxxiii]Creswell, J. D., Way, B. M., Eisenberger, N. I., & Lieberman, M. D. (2007). *Neural correlates of dispositional mindfulness during affect labeling*. Psychosomatic Medicine, 69(6), 560–565. https://doi.org/10.1097/PSY.0b013e3180f6171f

[xxxiv] Miller, E. K., & Cohen, J. D. (2001). *An integrative theory of prefrontal cortex function*. Annual Review of Neuroscience, 24, 167–202. https://doi.org/10.1146/annurev.neuro.24.1.167

[xxxv] Arnsten, A. F. T. (2009). *Stress signalling pathways that impair prefrontal cortex structure and function*. Nature Reviews Neuroscience, 10(6), 410–422. https://doi.org/10.1038/nrn2648

[xxxvi] McEwen, B. S., & Morrison, J. H. (2013). *The brain on stress: Vulnerability and plasticity of the prefrontal cortex over the life course*. Neuron, 79(1), 16–29. https://doi.org/10.1016/j.neuron.2013.06.028

[xxxvii] Eminem. (2002). *Lose yourself* [Song]. On *8 Mile: Music from and inspired by the motion picture*. Shady Records/Interscope Records.

[xxxviii] Teicher, M. H., & Samson, J. A. (2016). *Annual research review: Enduring neurobiological effects of childhood abuse and neglect*. Journal of Child Psychology and Psychiatry, 57(3), 241–266. https://doi.org/10.1111/jcpp.12507

[xxxix] Young (2011).

[xl] Settles, I. H., Buchanan, N. T., & Dotson, K. (2019). *Scrutinized but not recognized: (In)visibility and hypervisibility experiences of faculty of color*. Journal of Vocational Behavior, 113, 62–74. https://doi.org/10.1016/j.jvb.2018.06.003

[xli] Cokley, K., Smith, L., Bernard, D., Hurst, A., Jackson, S., Stone, S., & Roberts, D. (2017). *Impostor feelings as a moderator and mediator*

203

of the relationship between perceived discrimination and mental health among racial/ethnic minority college students. Journal of Counseling Psychology, 64(2), 141–154. https://doi.org/10.1037/cou0000198

[xlii] Clance (1978), 241–247.

[xliii] Tulshyan, R., & Burey, J. (2021). *Stop telling women they have imposter syndrome.* Harvard Business Review. https://hbr.org/2021/02/stop-telling-women-they-have-imposter-syndrome

[xliv] Fetterolf, J. C., & Eagly, A. H. (2011). *Do women expect to be leaders? The role of gender and leadership self-efficacy.* Psychology of Women Quarterly, 35(4), 507–518. https://doi.org/10.1177/0361684311410254

[xlv] Thomas, D. A., & Ely, R. J. (1996). *Making differences matter: A new paradigm for managing diversity.* Harvard Business Review. https://hbr.org/1996/09/making-differences-matter-a-new-paradigm-for-managing-diversity

[xlvi] Bowlby, J. (1969). *Attachment and Loss: Volume I. Attachment.* Basic Books.

[xlvii] Mikulincer, M., & Shaver, P. R. (2007). *Attachment in Adulthood: Structure, Dynamics, and Change.* Guilford Press.

[xlviii] Zanchetta, M., & Alessandri, G. (2021). Insecure Attachment and Impostor Phenomenon: A Mediation Model. *Personality and Individual Differences,* 181, 111071. https://doi.org/10.1016/j.paid.2021.111071

[xlix] Mikulincer (2007).

[l] Zeidner, M., & Matthews, G. (2000). *Intelligence and academic performance: From psychometrics to the developmental perspective of emotional intelligence.* In R. Bar-On & J. D. A. Parker (Eds.), *The Handbook of Emotional Intelligence* (pp. 215–243). Jossey-Bass.

[li] Gilbert, P. (2009). *The compassionate mind: A new approach to life's challenges.* New Harbinger Publications.

[lii] Crenshaw, K. (1989). *Demarginalizing the intersection of race and sex: A Black feminist critique of antidiscrimination doctrine, feminist theory and antiracist politics.* University of Chicago Legal Forum, 1989(1), Article 8

[liii] Cho, S., Crenshaw, K. W., & McCall, L. (2013). *Toward a field of intersectionality studies: Theory, applications, and praxis.* Signs: Journal of Women in Culture and Society, 38(4), 785–810. https://doi.org/10.1086/669608

[liv] Nadal, K. L., Griffin, K. E., Wong, Y., Hamit, S., & Rasmus, M. (2014). *The impact of racial microaggressions on mental health: Counseling implications for clients of color.* Journal of Counseling & Development, 92(1), 57–66. https://doi.org/10.1002/j.1556-6676.2014.00130.x

[lv] Tulshyan (2021).

[lvi] Cuddy, A. (2015). *Presence: Bringing Your Boldest Self to Your Biggest Challenges.* Little, Brown and Company.

[lvii] Greengross, G. (2013). Humor and the Big Five personality traits: Evidence for a relation between humor styles and openness to experience, extraversion, and agreeableness. *Personality and Individual Differences,* 54(4), 551–556. https://doi.org/10.1016/j.paid.2012.11.022

[lviii] Gilbert, P. (2010). *Compassion Focused Therapy: Distinctive Features.* Routledge

[lix] Burns, D. D. (1980). *Feeling Good: The New Mood Therapy.* William Morrow.

[lx] Beck, J. S. (2011). *Cognitive Behavior Therapy: Basics and Beyond* (2nd ed.). Guilford Press.

[lxi] Neff, K. D. (2011). *Self-Compassion: The Proven Power of Being Kind to Yourself.* William Morrow.

[lxii] Pennebaker, J. W., & Smyth, J. M. (2016). *Opening Up by Writing It Down: How Expressive Writing Improves Health and Eases Emotional Pain* (3rd ed.). Guilford Press.

[lxiii] Clance (1978), 241–247.

[lxiv]Young (2011).

[lxv] Clance (1978), 241–247.

[lxvi] American Psychological Association. (2019). *Burnout and stress: Causes, symptoms and prevention.*

[lxvii] Young, (2011).

[lxviii] Deci, E. L., & Ryan, R. M. (2000). The "what" and "why" of goal pursuits: Human needs and the self-determination of behavior. *Psychological Inquiry*, 11(4), 227–268.

www.ingramcontent.com/pod-product-compliance
Lightning Source LLC
Chambersburg PA
CBHW060144130626
46556CB00006B/2488